The Subtalar Joint

Editor

J. KENT ELLINGTON

FOOT AND ANKLE CLINICS

www.foot.theclinics.com

Consulting Editor
MARK S. MYERSON

June 2015 • Volume 20 • Number 2

ELSEVIER

1600 John F. Kennedy Boulevard • Suite 1800 • Philadelphia, Pennsylvania, 19103-2899

http://www.theclinics.com

FOOT AND ANKLE CLINICS Volume 20, Number 2
June 2015 ISSN 1083-7515, ISBN-13: 978-0-323-38886-3

Editor: Jennifer Flynn-Briggs
Developmental Editor: Meredith Clinton

Foot and Ankle Clinics (ISSN 1083-7515) is published quarterly by Elsevier, Inc., 360 Park Avenue South, New York, NY 10010-1710. Months of issue are March, June, September, and December. Periodicals postage paid at New York, NY, and additional mailing offices. Subscription price per year is $315.00 (US individuals), $421.00 (US institutions), $155.00 (US students), $360.00 (Canadian individuals), $506.00 (Canadian institutions), $215.00 (Canadian students), $460.00 (international individuals), $506.00 (international institutions), and $215.00 (international students). To receive student/resident rate, orders must be accompanied by name of affiliated institution, date of term, and the *signature* of program/residency coordinator on institution letterhead. Orders will be billed at individual rate until proof of status is received. Foreign air speed delivery is included in all *Clinics* subscription prices. All prices are subject to change without notice. **POSTMASTER:** Send address changes to *Foot and Ankle Clinics*, Elsevier Health Sciences Division, Subscription Customer Service, 3251 Riverport Lane, Maryland Heights, MO 63043. **Customer Service: 1-800-654-2452 (US and Canada). From outside of the United States and Canada, call 314-447-8871. Fax: 314-447-8029. E-mail: JournalsCustomerService-usa@ elsevier.com (for print support); JournalsOnlineSupport-usa@elsevier.com (for online support).**

Reprints. For copies of 100 or more, of articles in this publication, please contact the Commercial Reprints Department, Elsevier Inc., 360 Park Avenue South, New York, NY 10010-1710. Tel.: 212-633-3874; Fax: 212-633-3820; E-mail: reprints@elsevier.com.

Contributors

CONSULTING EDITOR

MARK S. MYERSON, MD
Director, The Institute for Foot and Ankle Reconstruction, Mercy Medical Center, Baltimore, Maryland

EDITOR

J. KENT ELLINGTON, MD, MS
OrthoCarolina, Foot and Ankle Institute, Charlotte, North Carolina

AUTHORS

MICHAEL AYNARDI, MD
Department of Orthopaedic Surgery, Rothman Institute of Orthopaedics, Thomas Jefferson University Hospital, Philadelphia, Pennsylvania

RAHUL BANERJEE, MD
Department of Orthopaedics, Advent Orthopaedics, Plano, Texas

STEPHEN F. CONTI, MD
Orthopaedic Foot and Ankle Fellowship Program, University of Pittsburgh, Pittsburgh, Pennsylvania

J. KENT ELLINGTON, MD, MS
OrthoCarolina, Foot and Ankle Institute, Charlotte, North Carolina

JAMES F. FLYNN, MD
Former Fellow; Orthopaedic Foot and Ankle Fellowship Program, University of Pittsburgh, Pittsburgh, Pennsylvania

ERIC GIZA, MD
Associate Professor; Chief, Foot and Ankle Surgery, Department of Orthopaedic Surgery, UC Davis Medical Center, Sacramento, California

JENS GORONZY, MD
Resident, Foot and Ankle Section, University Center for Orthopaedics and Traumatology, University Hospital Carl Gustav Carus, Dresden, Germany

CARL T. HASSELMAN, MD
Orthopaedic Foot and Ankle Fellowship Program, University of Pittsburgh, Pittsburgh, Pennsylvania

BEAT HINTERMANN, MD
Department of Orthopaedic Surgery, Kantonsspital Baselland, Liestal, Switzerland

MACALUS V. HOGAN, MD
Orthopaedic Foot and Ankle Fellowship Program, University of Pittsburgh, Pittsburgh, Pennsylvania

J. BENJAMIN JACKSON III, MD
Department of Orthopaedics, University of South Carolina, Columbia, South Carolina

LANCE JACOBSON, MD
Department of Orthopaedics, University of Utah, Salt Lake City, Utah

ALEX J. KLINE, MD
Orthopaedic Foot and Ankle Fellowship Program, University of Pittsburgh, Pittsburgh, Pennsylvania

MARKUS KNUPP, MD
Department of Orthopaedic Surgery, Kantonsspital Baselland, Liestal, Switzerland

CHRISTOPHER KREULEN, MD
Assistant Professor, Department of Orthopaedic Surgery, UC Davis Medical Center, Sacramento, California

TAMARA HORN LANG, PhD
Department of Orthopaedic Surgery, Kantonsspital Baselland, Liestal, Switzerland

ROBERT LOPEZ-BEN, MD
Clinical Professor, Department of Radiology, University of North Carolina School of Medicine at Charlotte; Staff Radiologist, Charlotte Radiology, Charlotte, North Carolina

ERNESTO MACEIRA, MD
Consultant in Orthopaedic Surgery, Associate Professor of Orthopaedic Surgery, Faculty of Medicine, Universidad Europea Madrid; Orthopaedic Foot and Ankle Unit, Orthopaedic and Trauma Department, Hospital Universitario Quirón Madrid, Madrid, Spain

MANUEL MONTEAGUDO, MD
Consultant in Orthopaedic Surgery, Associate Professor of Orthopaedic Surgery, Faculty of Medicine, Universidad Europea Madrid; Orthopaedic Foot and Ankle Unit, Orthopaedic and Trauma Department, Hospital Universitario Quirón Madrid, Madrid, Spain

VINCENT S. MOSCA, MD
Chief; Pediatric Orthopedic Surgeon, Pediatric Foot and Ankle Service, Seattle Children's Hospital; Professor of Orthopedics, Department of Orthopaedics and Sports Medicine, University of Washington School of Medicine, Seattle, Washington

MARK S. MYERSON, MD
Director, The Institute for Foot and Ankle Reconstruction, Mercy Medical Center, Baltimore, Maryland

FLORIAN NICKISCH, MD
Department of Orthopaedics, University of Utah, Salt Lake City, Utah

DAVID I. PEDOWITZ, MD
Assistant Professor Orthopaedic Surgery, Rothman Institute of Orthopaedics, Thomas Jefferson University Hospital, Philadelphia, Pennsylvania

JULIAN RÖHM, MD
Department of Orthopaedic Surgery, Kantonsspital Baselland, Liestal, Switzerland

STEVEN M. RAIKIN, MD
Director, Foot and Ankle Service; Professor Orthopaedic Surgery, Rothman Institute of Orthopaedics, Thomas Jefferson University Hospital, Philadelphia, Pennsylvania

STEFAN RAMMELT, MD, PhD
Professor; Head, Foot and Ankle Section, University Center for Orthopaedics and Traumatology, University Hospital Carl Gustav Carus, Dresden, Germany

BRENT ROSTER, MD
Department of Orthopaedic Surgery, UC Davis Medical Center, Sacramento, California

ETTORE VULCANO, MD
The Institute for Foot and Ankle Reconstruction, Mercy Medical Center, Baltimore, Maryland

DANE K. WUKICH, MD
Orthopaedic Foot and Ankle Fellowship Program, University of Pittsburgh, Pittsburgh, Pennsylvania

LUKAS ZWICKY, MSc
Department of Orthopaedic Surgery, Kantonsspital Baselland, Liestal, Switzerland

Contents

Understanding subtalar joint biomechanics and pathomechanics provides a framework for understanding both common pathologic hindfoot and forefoot conditions and surgical planning. It is important to identify mechanical impairment and to define what mechanical effect is needed to change a pathologic condition. It is also important to know what the initial problem is and what the consequences are in terms of soft tissue or bony stress leading to peritalar injury. Whenever possible, one should try to operate to change pathomechanics and facilitate spontaneous repair of stressed structures.

Imaging of the subtalar joint can be challenging because of its complex planar anatomy. This article reviews the anatomy and common anatomic variants as seen with different imaging techniques. Although radiography remains the initial mode of imaging, computed tomography and MRI are frequently needed to better delineate the joint anatomy and improve the sensitivity and the specificity of detection of joint pathology. A short review of arthrographic techniques and various examples of imaging of common pathology involving this joint are also included.

Subtalar instability is a common clinical entity. Clinicians should have a high index of suspicion of this diagnosis in patients who have been diagnosed with chronic lateral ankle instability but have failed standard management and have continued pain in the sinus tarsi. As with ankle instability, nonoperative management is the initial mainstay of treatment. Operative management includes ligamentous reconstruction of key lateral stabilizers of the subtalar joint. Future research on this subject should be focused at improving diagnosis and recognition of this entity.

Subtalar dislocations make up 1-2% of all dislocations, about 75% of them being medial dislocations. Treatment consists of early reduction under adequate sedation. In cases of soft tissue interposition or locked dislocations, open reduction is warranted. More than 60% of subtalar dislocations are associated with additional fractures, therefore a postreduction CT is recommended. Complications include avascular necrosis of the talus, infection, posttraumatic arthritis, chronic subtalar instability, and complex regional pain syndrome with delayed reduction. The prognosis of purely ligamentous injuries is excellent after early reduction. Negative prognostic factors include lateral and open dislocations, total talar dislocations, and associated fractures.

wound healing problems occur less frequently. Avascular necrosis of the talus is a rare but serious complication, although frequency seems to be independent of the approach chosen. Clinical studies showed no increased morbidity when comparing the medial to the lateral approach.

FOOT AND ANKLE CLINICS

RELATED INTEREST

Orthopedic Clinics of North America
April 2015 (Vol. 46, No. 2)
Asif M. Ilyas, Shital N. Parikh, Saqib Rehman, Giles R. Scuderi and
Felasfa M. Wodajo, *Editors*

Preface

The Subtalar Joint: It Is More Complicated Than You Think

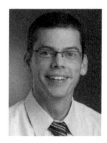

J. Kent Ellington, MD, MS
Editor

Understanding the subtalar joint is extremely important in order to grasp the complexity of the foot. The anatomy and biomechanics are crucial to the function of the hindfoot, ankle, midfoot, and even forefoot. This issue provides expertise in areas ranging from anatomy, radiology, biomechanics, congenital and acquired conditions, and treatment options of the subtalar joint. Proper history and physical examination, along with imaging, are important to diagnose and appropriately treat the patient. Subtleties are important, and attention to detail can be the difference in a satisfied patient versus a poor outcome.

J. Kent Ellington, MD, MS
OrthoCarolina
Foot and Ankle Institute
2001 Vail Ave, Ste 200Bane
Charlotte, NC 28207, USA

E-mail address:
kentellingtonfx@gmail.com

Foot Ankle Clin N Am 20 (2015) xi
http://dx.doi.org/10.1016/j.fcl.2015.03.001
1083-7515/15/$ – see front matter © 2015 Published by Elsevier Inc.

Subtalar Anatomy and Mechanics

Ernesto Maceira, MD[a,b], Manuel Monteagudo, MD[a,b],*

KEYWORDS

- Subtalar joint • Mechanics • Pathomechanics • Talus • Calcaneus • Peritalar
- Osteotomy

KEY POINTS

- Sinus tarsi and its ligaments are late phylogenetic structures, typical of human feet that are prepared for bipedal position.
- To understand how the peritalar complex works, it may be assumed that the subtalar joint (STJ) axis is a single axis of a mitered hinge.
- By supinating the STJ during the second and third rockers of gait, the foot is converted from a shock-absorbing structure into a rigid lever, which provides the foot with the greatest mechanical efficiency for pushing off.
- In both pronatory and supinatory syndromes, reducing the mechanical stress on the injured area will promote healing and restore flexibility and strength of the involved tissues.
- Both nonoperative and operative management strategies regarding the STJ should aim to restore balance between the external and the internal moments, thus reducing tissue stress.

INTRODUCTION

There is ambiguity in the use of the term "subtalar joint" regarding the involvement of the talus, the calcaneus, and the navicular. Herein, the "subtalar joint" is referred to as synonymous with the talocalcaneal joint. The subtalar joint (STJ) is designed to quickly change from a flexible shock-absorbing structure to a rigid propulsive one. Function makes form. The embryology, anatomy, and mechanics of the STJ are reviewed. This article does not attempt to simply review the available literature on STJ anatomy and mechanics but instead tries to make STJ function easy to understand for the clinician. A correlation between mechanics and surgery around the STJ is also presented.

The authors have nothing to disclose.
[a] Universidad Europea Madrid, s/n, Calle Tajo, 28670 Villaviciosa de Odón, Madrid, Spain;
[b] Orthopaedic Foot and Ankle Unit, Orthopaedic and Trauma Department, Hospital Universitario Quirón Madrid, Calle Diego de Velázquez n°1, 28223 Pozuelo de Alarcón, Madrid, Spain
* Corresponding author. Hospital Universitario, Quirón Madrid, Calle Diego de Velázquez n°1, 28223 Pozuelo de Alarcón, Madrid, Spain.
E-mail address: mmontyr@yahoo.com

EMBRYOLOGY

Tarsal bones can be recognized as early as the 14 mm crown-rump (C-R) (43 days). Between the 14 and 17 mm C-R, the tarsus is shown as a mesenchymal structure located in the distal portion of the bones of the lower extremity.[1] A small artery, which appears at the 14 mm C-R and disappears at 18 mm C-R, divides the posterior tarsus into the talus medially and the calcaneus laterally.[2] At around 27 mm C-R (55 days), the sustentaculum tali arises and the talus is placed almost completely over the calcaneus. At 34 mm C-R (61 days), the posterior STJ surface is easily identified. At 110 mm C-R (16 weeks), the sinus tarsi is visualized and the nerve and vascular arch within the sinus tarsi are evident. Most authors consider the sinus tarsi artery as an anastomosis through the sinus tarsi between the plantar and dorsal systems.[3] Ligaments at the sinus tarsi do not develop until the fetal stage is advanced (40 mm C-R) and possibly play a role in the straightening of the foot within the first weeks of the fetal stage. Sinus tarsi and its ligaments are late phylogenetic structures, typical of human feet that are prepared for bipedal position (**Fig. 1**).

DESCRIPTIVE ANATOMY
The Talus and Talar Articular Facets

The talus is covered by articular cartilage on more than 60% of its surface and has no muscle insertions. Thus, the talus moves because peritalar structures move. The STJ usually has 3 articular facets on the inferior part of the talus and the superior part of the calcaneus. The posterior facet is the largest and forms a saddlelike joint under the talus, with a concave shape in the long axis. There is considerable variation in shape and size of the facets. The posterior facet is separated from the anterior and middle facets. The anterior and middle facets are often continuous.

The Calcaneus and Calcaneus Articular Facets

Two or 3 articular facets mirror those of the talus. The posterior facet is located in the middle third of the calcaneus. The anterior third of the calcaneus supports the anterior and middle facets. The calcaneal surface contributes to the formation of the "sustentaculum tali" over which the talus leans. The sustentaculum tali provides a sliding surface for the posterior tibial tendon, the flexor hallucis longus tendon, and the flexor

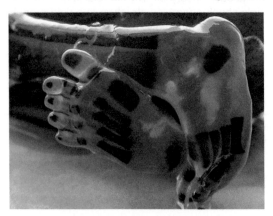

Fig. 1. Ossification of the forefoot takes place earlier than that at mid- and hindfoot. Alizarin stained fetus from the Collection of the Department of Anatomy and Embryology 1. Faculty of Medicine, Universidad Complutense de Madrid, Spain.

digitorum tendon. The classical description by Basmajian[4] and Testut and Latarjet[5] consider 3 types of anterior STJs (1) with a more or less ovoid shape; (2) in the form of a bean, narrowed in the medial part; and (3) completely divided in 2 parts. Viladot examined 100 calcanei of cadavers and found 42% of ovoid forms, 22% of bean forms, and 36% divided into 2 parts.[1] The anterior STJ also contributes to the formation of the coxa pedis, along with the posterior surface of the navicular, the calcaneonavicular ligament (spring ligament), and the fibrocartilago navicularis.[6]

Sinus Tarsi and Ligaments

The sinus tarsi is situated between the talocalcaneonavicular joint anteriorly and the posterior talocalcaneal joint posteriorly. The wide anterolateral part of this conical cavity is the sinus tarsi itself, whereas the narrower posteromedial part is known as the canalis tarsi.[7]

There is a great variability of descriptions about shape, orientation, and location of the sinus tarsi ligaments.[8–12] Smith was the first to describe 3 different ligaments within the sinus tarsi that settled consensus from the literature[13]:

1. Posterior band of the interosseous talocalcaneal ligament (also known as the "ligament of the tarsal canal," the "ligamentum talocalcaneale interosseum," the "interosseous talocalcaneal ligament," the "ligament of Farabeuf," the "cruciate ligament of the tarsus," the "axial ligament," or the "oblique astragalocalcaneal ligament").
2. Anterior band of the interosseous talocalcaneal ligament (also known as the "cervical ligament or ligamentum cervicis," the "anterior lateral talocalcaneus ligament," the "external talus calcaneal ligament," the "interosseous anterior ligament," or the "ligament of Fick").
3. Inferior extensor retinaculum (also known as the "cruciform ligaments," the "cruciatum-cruris ligaments," the "frondiform ligament," or the "ligament of Retzius").

GEOMETRICAL PARAMETERS OF THE SUBTALAR JOINT; ARTICULAR SURFACES, AXIS OF MOTION

Articular surfaces of the STJ are much like sections of cylinders.[14] STJ is formed by 2 cylindrical joints; the posterior STJ has a concave facet at the talus, whereas the anterior STJ has a concave facet at the calcaneus, the latter being usually the union of the anterior and middle calcaneal facets. A simple mechanical model of the STJ is depicted in **Fig. 2**.

When moving an anatomic specimen, it may be appreciated that there is permanent contact between the articular facets throughout its full range of motion, so that the articular contact pattern is through gliding, as opposed to a rolling contact pattern in which one side of the joint would open while the joint moves toward the opposite side. By definition, the axis of motion of a gliding contact pattern joint, when one of the surfaces is convex, passes through the geometric center of the convex surface.[15] The center of rotation of the STJ passes through the geometric center of the talar head and the geometric center of the calcaneal posterior surface or thalamus. The axis of motion lies perpendicular to the anatomically longer diameter of the facets. The STJ axis shows an inclination from dorsal, medial, and anterior to plantar, lateral, and posterior in the anatomic position, as described by Henke.[16] Because it is a triplane axis, motion around the STJ axis occurs simultaneously in all 3 reference planes.

The STJ is a single-axis joint that acts as a mitered hinge connecting the talus and the calcaneus. Should the STJ axis be inclined 45° from transverse, a simple torque converter is created, meaning rotation of the vertical member is coupled to equal rotation of the horizontal member. A vertically aligned STJ axis (over 45°), such as that of a cavus foot, causes less rotation of the horizontal segment for a given rotation of the vertical one.[17] A more horizontally aligned axis (as in a flatfoot) causes a greater rotation of

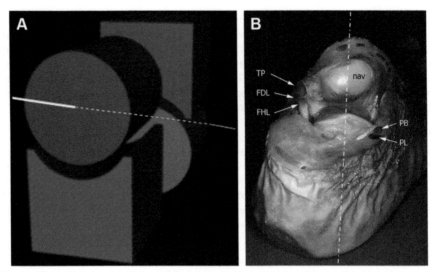

Fig. 2. (*A*) A simple mechanical model of the subtalar joint. Two rigid bodies articulating with each other by a pair of cylindrical joints with a convex and a concave facet. Motion between them takes place by means of a gliding contact pattern, about an axis that passes through the geometric centers of the convex surfaces: the talar head in the anterior part and the thalamus of the calcaneus in the posterior part. (*B*) Mechanics of the STJ on weight-bearing conditions include complex motion to allow for axial rotation of the leg on the transverse plane over a stable foot. A single-axis joint model could not work in real life but provides us with an approach to understanding subtalar function. The acetabulum pedis allows for the talar head to ride on or beside the anterior process of the calcaneus. When the leg is externally rotated, the medial column lies on the lateral column at the midtarsal joint. When the foot is pronated, the talar head points medially in the acetabulum pedis and the leg is internally rotated. Subtalar joint axis is represented by the dotted yellow line. The solid red lines represent the shape of the calcaneal subtalar joint facets, the anterior being concave upwards and the posterior convex upwards. TP, tibialis posterior; FDL, flexor digitorum longus; FHL, flexor hallucis longus; PB, peroneus brevis; PL, peroneus longus, nav, navicular.

the horizontal member for a given rotation of the vertical member. Thus, individuals with a flatfoot deformity, that is, a more horizontal STJ axis, show greater supination/pronation (motion at the longitudinal axis of the horizontal segment) for a given external/internal rotation of the vertical segment. Considering motion on a triplane axis, its amplitude will be greater in the plane that lies closer to the perpendicular plane to the axis; the corresponding coordinate plane is referred to as dominant. Kapandji[18] compared STJ motion to that of a cardan drive. The talus is the middle piece of a cardan transmission between the foot and the leg. Manter[19] studied STJ motion in 16 cadaveric specimens and found the axis runs in a downward, outward, and backward direction, making an angle as viewed from the side of about 42° with the transverse plane and as viewed from above of about 16° with the sagittal plane. Isman and Inman[20] pointed out the variability in STJ axis alignment. Their study on 46 cadaveric legs found that, in the transverse plane, the axis deviated 23° medial to the long axis of the foot with a range of 4° to 47°, whereas in the sagittal plane, the axis was close to 41°, with a range of 21° to 69°. Van Langelaan[21] performed a quantitative stereo-photogrammetric study of the STJ. He described its axis as a mobile concept; motion at the tarsal joints can be described to happen around a bundle of discrete axes (a helical axis).

Quantitative analysis of motion at the tarsal joints can be influenced by the fact of considering the axis to be a simple static axis or a moving helical axis, but to understand how the peritalar complex works, it may be assumed that the STJ axis is a single axis of a mitered hinge.

MOVEMENTS AT THE SUBTALAR JOINT: OPEN VERSUS CLOSED KINETIC CHAIN

One of the properties of a hinge joint is that rotation always remains in the same plane: motion occurs in a plane perpendicular to the hinge's axis.[15] When considering the talocalcaneal joint alone, it has one degree of freedom: a single coordinate is enough to describe the position and alignment of the joint. Pronation is a triplane motion consisting of simultaneous movements of abduction on the transverse plane, dorsiflexion on the sagittal plane, and eversion on the coronal plane. Supination is a triplane motion combining adduction around a vertical axis, plantarflexion through a transverse axis, and inversion on the longitudinal axis. In the European literature, the terms inversion and eversion refer to the compound motion.[18,22,23] In normal conditions, two-thirds of the STJ range of motion correspond to supination and one-third correspond to pronation. Normal passive STJ range of motion is around 30°, although 10° of supination and 5° of pronation allow for a normal gait.

The sagittal plane is the least dominant plane in STJ motion so that STJ impairments may not affect progression of gait, which depends on sagittal plane motion. Hicks[15] described how several of his colleagues considered STJ motion to be insignificant. The levers that form the STJ are very short. All these facts make the STJ a nonessential joint for gait and posture (as long as it is properly aligned).[24] It is unlikely that STJ joint replacement may become a sensible procedure, because subtalar arthrodesis works quite well when compared with fusion of the ankle or the talonavicular joints.

During foot pronation/supination, the largest amount of motion occurs at the talonavicular joint followed by the talocalcaneal joint; in the latter, motion occurs mainly by supination.[25,26] Fusion of the talonavicular joint completely blocks motion at the STJ, but not oppositely: fusion of the STJ allows for significant motion at the neighboring joints.[27]

During pronation, the sinus tarsi closes because the lateral process of the talus glides anteriorly toward the prethalamic surface of the calcaneus. During foot supination, the sinus tarsi opens. This feature is important to consider during hindfoot surgery; while the patient is lying down and the surgeon cannot see the actual alignment of the hindfoot, a closed sinus tarsi means the STJ is everted, whereas an opened sinus means the STJ is inverted. In certain procedures, it is advisable to set the STJ in valgus (ie, tibiotalocalcaneal fusion), while in others it is advisable to set the STJ alignment in varus (ie, STJ arthroereisis for flatfoot) (**Fig. 3**).

Open Versus Closed Kinetic Chain

The motion pattern of the STJ joint is completely different in open or closed kinetic chain conditions. STJ motion in the open kinetic chain has been classically described by the anatomists. It takes place when there is no external force opposing foot motion. In this situation, the muscles have an origin at the proximal end, and their distal end or insertion is the point that moves when muscle contraction takes place. During open kinetic chain motion, a muscle acts on the joints it crosses. Depending on the anatomic relations of the tendons crossing the STJ, they can be grouped into invertors and evertors (**Fig. 4**). The tendons inverting the STJ (posterior tibialis, flexor digitorum longus, and flexor hallucis longus) are those that cross the STJ medial to its axis, whereas the evertors run laterally with respect to the STJ axis.

The posterior tibial muscle is the more powerful subtalar invertor, because it has the longest moment arm and the largest physiologic cross-section.[28] The tibialis anterior muscle is a strong subtalar invertor and ankle dorsiflexor; its action on the STJ

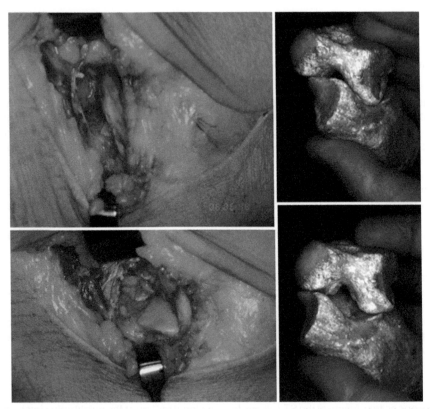

Fig. 3. The sinus tarsi closes when the STJ is pronated. Conversely, it opens when the STJ is inverted. This is an important morphologic feature for the surgeon to be aware of, since during surgery there is no way to accurately assess real leg-foot-ground alignment.

depends on the relative position of the foot because the tendon moment arm is variable. The extensor hallucis longus shows a similar behavior on the STJ; it is an ankle dorsiflexor, but may exert supination or pronation on the STJ depending on the initial position of the foot. The extensor digitorum longus is an STJ pronator, together with the peroneus tertius. Ankle dorsiflexion moment during the swing phase is provided by the tibialis anterior, the long toe extensors, and the peroneus tertius. The action of the tibialis anterior must be counterbalanced by the extensor digitorum longus and the peroneus tertius to properly align the foot on the coronal plane; otherwise, a net inverting moment would result at the STJ in the initial contact. Both the peroneus brevis and the peroneus longus are STJ pronators and ankle plantar flexors in open kinetic chain contraction. The triceps suralis is an STJ invertor because in the normally aligned foot, the insertion of the Achilles tendon on the calcaneal tuberosity is medial to the STJ axis.

However, muscle action during closed kinetic chain conditions is completely different. When the foot supports the body weight, its motion is restrained by the external moments derived from the inertial forces, gravity, and ground reaction forces. If the internal moment generated by any muscle acting on a joint is lower than the external moments acting on that joint, the fixed end of the muscle will be the distal one and it will be the proximal end that moves. In closed kinetic chain conditions, the force applied is not great enough to overcome the resistance. For instance, the soleus muscle in open kinetic chain conditions is an ankle plantar flexor, but during the second

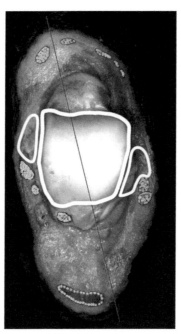

Fig. 4. Tendons crossing the STJ medially with respect to the axis are open kinetic chain in-vertors, while those crossing the joint laterally are evertors. Some of them may behave as invertors or evertors depending on the relative position of the foot with respect to the leg when muscle action is considered. Red line represents subtalar joint axis.

rocker (plantigrade support) of the gait cycle, it stops the forward rotation of the tibia, thus extending the knee because of the coupled action with the inertial force derived from body progression. Therefore, the muscle is acting on a joint it does not cross and its fixed end is the distal one. During the propulsive period (third rocker), the triceps will be able to elevate the body center of mass because the center of mass is progressing forward and the vertical component of the external forces is lower; the plantar flexor ankle moment exceeds the external dorsiflexor moment at the ankle. If the ground is not firm enough, part of the muscle force is spent in deforming the ground instead of providing for propulsive power, thus resulting in fatigue. On a firm ground during closed kinetic chain, the posterior tibial tendon will not be able to produce plantar flexion, nor internal rotation or inversion of the foot, but it will instead push the medial malleolus forward, providing an external rotation moment on the leg (**Fig. 5**). Because of the anatomic arrangement of the ankle mortise, with the medial malleolus being anterior with respect to the lateral one, the external rotation of the leg is transmitted to the talus, moving its head laterally (**Fig. 6**). The anterior articular facet of the calcaneus as seen from the front represents a curved slope that enables the talar head to ride on it when the leg is externally rotated. The navicular follows the talar head, so the medial column is placed over the lateral column. By this active mechanism, the foot converts into a rigid structure for propulsion, a stiff lever to allow for the Achilles-calcaneus-plantar system to push off. During the third rocker, the body weight is transmitted to the ground from the tibia to the talus, navicular, cuneiforms, and the first 3 metatarsals supporting axial compression with the Achilles-calcaneal-plantar system supporting tensile stress. Failure to achieve external rotation of the leg during the second rocker will not externally rotate the talus, thus: (1) the medial column will suffer medial plantar

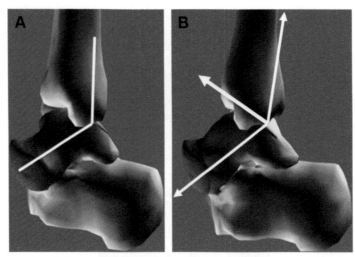

Fig. 5. During weight-bearing (closed kinetic chain), the foot is not free to move as a consequence of muscle contraction unless the internal moments exceed the external moments. The tibialis posterior tendon is not able to produce a net effect of plantarflexion, adduction, and inversion of the foot, but instead it pushes the medial malleolus forward thus providing the leg with an external rotation moment. (*A*) Resting position; (*B*) tibialis posterior action. Tibialis posterior contraction under close kinetic chain conditions generates a resulting force which pushes the medial malleolus forward thus externally rotating the leg. Arrowheads represent force vectors produced by the tibialis posterior tendon.

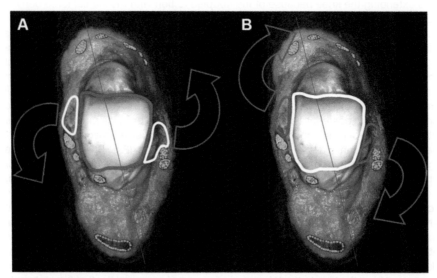

Fig. 6. The malleolar arrangement at the ankle mortise, with the medial malleolus anterior with respect to the lateral malleolus on the transverse plane, makes internal rotation of the talus being transmitted to the leg (*A*) and external rotation of the leg transmitted to the talus (*B*), but the reverse is not true.

tensile stress for which it is not prepared to cope with, and (2) the force provided by the Achilles tendon will not act on the metatarsophalangeal break line but on the midtarsal joint, contributing to the pronatory deforming forces.

In static stance, the STJ will move if axial rotation at the leg or the foot is initiated. The internal rotation of the leg must be necessarily coupled to foot pronation, and the external rotation of the leg must be coupled to supination of the foot. This is the function of the peritalar complex as a cardan drive, the talus being its middle segment. The talus does not receive muscle insertions, so it moves as the consequence of motion of its neighboring segments.

Rotation about a vertical axis is also noticed in one-leg balancing; when the foot tends to supinate, the leg rotates laterally, and when the foot tends to pronate, the leg rotates medially.[15] By this chain of actions, the femur laterally rotates at the hip joint when the big toe is lifted off the ground. In the absence of talo-calcaneo-navicular action, these movements do not occur and one-leg balancing is impossible.

CLINICAL ASSESSMENT OF THE SUBTALAR JOINT AXIS

The spatial location of the STJ axis is quite variable. Kirby[29] described a clinical method to assess the projection of the STJ axis on the sole of the foot during planti-grade support. It is based on the fact that a force applied directly on a system axis of rotation will produce no turning motion because the moment of that force is zero. If the force is applied at a distance from the axis, it will produce rotation. With the patient lying prone, the examiner places the ankle joint in neutral by applying dorsiflexion from the lateral metatarsal heads. The sole of the foot is then pushed upwards at different points of the plantar surface. "If the thumb pushing on the plantar foot is medial to the subtalar joint axis, then subtalar joint supination occurs, and if the thumb pushes lateral to the subtalar joint axis, then *subtalar joint pronation occurs.*"[30] If there is pronation or supination, the STJ axis is not projected on that point (**Fig. 7**). Conversely, when the examiner pushes just on the projected axis, both the patient and the examiner will feel an upward displacement with no turning effect at the foot. The point is marked and the operation is repeated at another level (anterior/posterior). The resulting marks will allow the examiner to draw a line, which represents the projection of the STJ axis on the transverse plane. The normally aligned axis runs from the lateral aspect of the posterior heel to the first metatarsal head or the first intermetatarsal space. The authors do not attempt to use this method for quantitative assessment but instead to simply make an estimation of whether a foot will tend to supinate or pronate in response to ground reaction forces. A foot that shows supination while walking will present an STJ axis with a lateral deviation. This clinical test for STJ axis placement can be also used for intraoperative assessment of STJ varus or valgus.[31]

HOW DOES THE SUBTALAR JOINT INFLUENCE THE STRUCTURAL STIFFNESS OF THE FOOT?

From a morphologic point of view, the plantar vault is the result of the bicolumnar structure of the foot. During static stance, both columns lie distally at the same level, but at the proximal end (in the midtarsal joint), the talar column lies over the calcaneal column. The main neurovascular bundle of the foot is protected by the presence of the plantar arch. From a mechanical point of view, the plantar vault ensures the foot can behave both as a compliant bag of loose bones (pronated foot) and as a rigid lever (supinated foot).

By placing the proximal end of both columns one over the other (foot supination), the calcaneal foot protects the foot against intrinsic dorsiflexion. The calcaneo-cuboid joint is well designed to resist dorsiflexing moments, because of its shape and strong

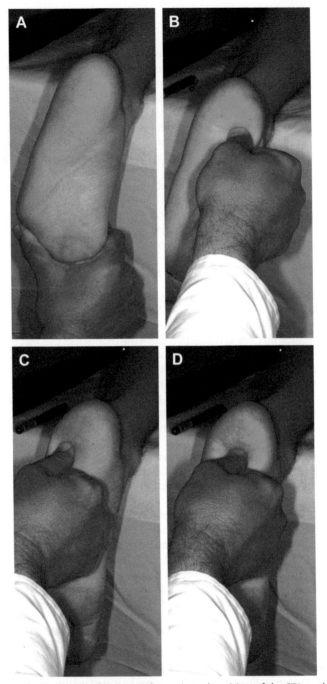

Fig. 7. Kirby's palpation method to assess the projected position of the STJ on the transverse plane during static stance or mid second rocker. With the patient prone, the foot is held from the lateral distal metatarsals to reach ankle neutral position (*A*). The examiner pushes the sole of the foot upwards at a point of the heel, producing a turning motion of the foot into supination (*B*) or pronation (*C*), depending on whether the chosen points lie medial or lateral to the STJ axis. When the palpated point is just under the projection of the axis on the sole of the foot, both the patient and the examiner will feel a pushing-up effect instead of any turning motion at the foot (*D*).

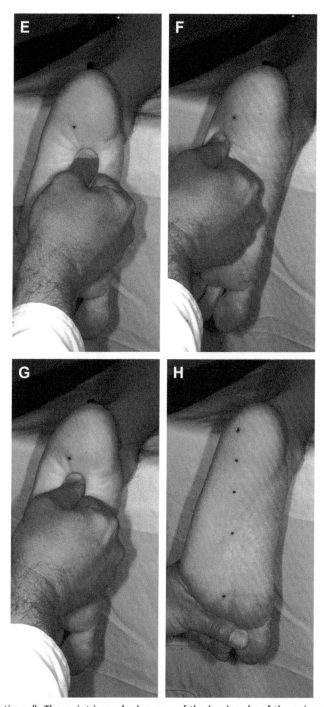

Fig. 7. (*continued*). The point is marked as one of the landmarks of the axis projection (*E*) and the same operation is performed at another level (*F, G*). Finally, the marked points allow us to estimate the location of the projected axis (*H*), which usually runs from the posterior lateral portion of the heel to the first metatarsal head or first intermetatarsal space. The effect of the external forces will be pronating moments on the STJ for those acting lateral to the axis. This test is critical for orthotic design and may be useful in the study of certain patients that will undergo surgery.

plantar ligaments. When the calcaneo-cuboid joint is placed underneath the talonavicular joint, the latter is protected against dorsiflexing moments. The talonavicular joint is well prepared to resist compressive axial loading when the joint lies horizontal, during the propulsive phase. However, the talonavicular joint is not designed to cope with dorsiflexing moments while the joint lies vertically aligned, as it is during static stance and the second rocker (plantigrade support during the gait cycle) **(Fig. 8)**.

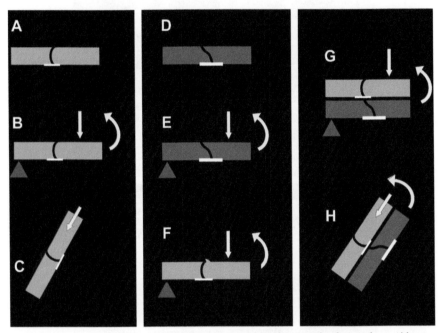

Fig. 8. The foot as a bi-columnar structure governed by the STJ. The foot is formed by two columns: the talar column and the calcaneal column. The talar column has a mobile enarthrodial joint at the midtarsal level, the talonavicular joint (A) which shows a curved shape and a relatively weak plantar spring ligament. The figure depicts a simplified joint with no real attachments. This type of joint is not well prepared to resist body weight (straight arrows) during the second rocker (B). It will easily collapse but, on the other hand, serve as a shock absorbing structure. The curved arrows represent action of the triceps suralis. The talar column is very well prepared to cope with axial compressive loading during the third rocker (C), while the foot is vertical on the ground. The calcaneal foot at the level of the midtarsal region has an ideal shape to oppose dorsiflexing moments, and is protected by the strongest ligament of the foot, the calcaneo-cuboid complex (D). Its anatomic arrangement is ideal to cope with second rocker and static stance stress (E). If the talar foot is asked to work as a calcaneal foot from the earlier stages of development, its form will adapt to that abnormal function developing a talar beak that actually resembles the shape of the calcaneo-cuboid joint (F). We understand the talar beak not as a common osteophyte but as an osseous adaptation. By the late second rocker, the ideal arrangement of both foot columns is that in which the talar foot overrides the lateral column, so that the latter prevents dorsiflexion at the talonavicular joint (G), which in turn will perfectly cope with the body weight axial loading while the medial column is vertically aligned (H). The picture in the right (I) shows how the STJ is the structure that allows for both columns to be arranged in a (pronated side to side) shock-absorbing structure or a (supinated medial column over lateral column) rigid lever display.

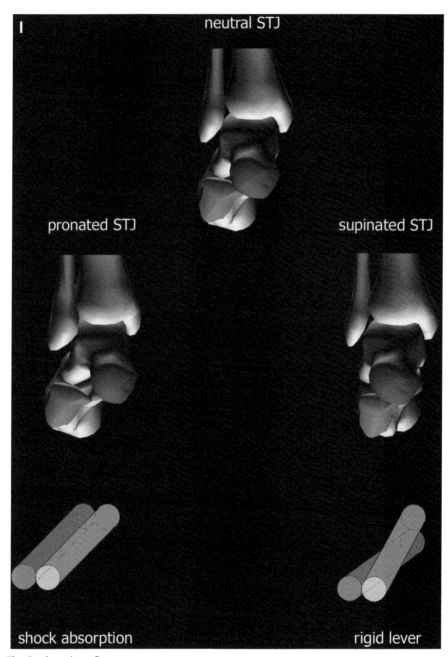

Fig. 8. (*continued*).

FORM AND FUNCTION OF THE PERITALAR COMPLEX: OSSEOUS ADAPTATION

By the end of the embryonic period, the mesenchymal tissue at the future joints must undergo a programmed necrotic process with no inflammatory response (apoptosis) to form the joint cavities. In at least 1% of the embryos, apoptosis may not take place, leading to the development of fibrous, chondral, or osseous union between the future tarsal bones. When a tarsal coalition develops, the cardan mechanism of the talo-calcaneo-navicular joint may get completely blocked and the ankle joint may be in the need to deal with the axial turning motion between the leg and the foot.[32] In such instances, the ankle joint shape may be spherical (ball-and-socket ankle) instead of cylindrical (conical) to allow for both plantar/dorsal flexion on the sagittal plane and inversion/eversion around the longitudinal axis at the same time (**Fig. 9**). The reason tarsal coalitions are usually associated with valgus deformity of the STJ remains unclear. Most of the patients with a tarsal coalition present with hindfoot valgus, unless there is a concomitant disease leading to subtalar varus. Although the longitudinal arch is usually flat in patients with tarsal coalition, it might be normal or show an increased height.

The talar beak is a prominence at the dorsal-lateral aspect of the talar head that appears as an osseous adaptation to long-term foot pronation. In the presence of a talar

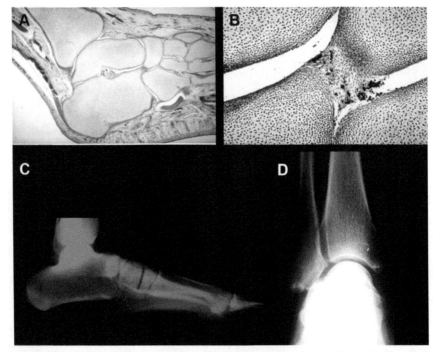

Fig. 9. (A) A sagittal section of a specimen at the late embryonic period/early fetal period. A close-up of the future calcaneo-navicular area shows dark necrotic cells without inflammatory response, taking place on the mesenchymal tissue. Apoptosis is a programmed cell death, necessary for joint cavitation among other developmental requirements (B). When this necrotic process fails to occur, a link will persist between two or more of the skeletal elements of the peritalar complex, producing a tarsal coalition. Depending on the remaining type of tissue, the coalition may be osseous (synostosis), cartilage (synchondrosis), or fibrous (synfibrosis or syndesmosis). (C) Shows a complex pantalar coalition in which subtalar motion is completely blocked. In such circumstances, axial torque conversion between the leg and the foot may take place at the ankle joint which copes simultaneously with the requirements of both the ankle and the STJ. This abnormal function creates an abnormal ball-and-socket shape (D). Histological sections from the Collection of the Department of Anatomy and Embryology 1. Faculty of Medicine, Universidad Complutense de Madrid, Spain.

beak, a tarsal coalition should be ruled out. However, the sign may be present in the foot with normal motion at the STJ as well. If the talonavicular joint is required to oppose to dorsiflexing moments from an early age, it may adapt itself morphologically to gain resistance to dorsiflexion. The curved articular surfaces would be intrinsically best prepared to resist dorsiflexion if there is a bony block limiting dorsiflexion of the talonavicular joint (see **Fig. 8**).

MECHANICAL DIAGNOSIS

The diagnosis of any mechanical impairment of the foot must be based on clinical examination and plain weight-bearing radiograph of both feet. Clinical examination must be performed in both non-weight-bearing and weight-bearing conditions (patient standing, sitting, and walking).

Assessment of Subtalar Joint Alignment in Weight-Bearing Radiographs

Because of a lack of repeatability, the authors do not routinely measure angles on the radiographs. They prefer to estimate bony alignment by the analysis of qualitative parameters, which they find to be reliable. Therefore, instead of collecting numbers, they can describe certain morphologic features that may present depending on foot alignment (**Table 1**).

A difference in the height of both ankle joints in the anteroposterior weight-bearing view suggests a relative STJ pronation (lower) or supination (higher). A few degrees in the talar inclination angle may be difficult to identify on the lateral weight-bearing radiographs, but a few millimeters of difference in the height of the tibiotalar joints is clearly seen in the anteroposterior view of both ankles. In the pronated foot, the ankle is internally rotated so the overlapping area between the tibia and fibula is reduced.

THE SUBTALAR JOINT DURING THE GAIT CYCLE: THE 3 GAIT ROCKERS

The "3 rockers" from gait analysis are referred to so as to understand the mechanics of the STJ.[33–35]

First Rocker (Heel Strike–Shock Absorption)

Pronation that occurs at initial heel contact is a passive mechanism that takes place because of the tibiocalcaneal desaxation. The calcaneal tuberosity should lie slightly lateral with respect to the projection of the tibial shaft, so that a pair of forces is formed between the ground reaction force and the body weight. The talar head turns medially and drags the ankle joint because of the disposition of the malleoli (medial malleolus is anterior and lateral is posterior). Internal rotation of the talus is well transmitted to the leg and external rotation of the leg is well transmitted to the talus because of the anatomic arrangement of the mortise (see **Fig. 6**). The initial contact is actually a hammer blow, as demonstrated by quantitative gait analysis. The butterfly diagram depicting the instant ground reaction force vector shows that it is pointing to the body center of mass, except for the loading response vector, which is vertically oriented, thus representing a free fall. In order for the hammer blow to be balanced, the head and the handle of the hammer must be aligned. If the head is displaced with respect to the shaft, an immediate turn to the opposite side will be produced after the impact (**Fig. 10**). Avoiding that turning effect is not achieved by holding the hammer stronger using both hands (increasing internal force), but rather by aligning head and shaft (reducing the external moment arm).

Table 1
Radiology of the STJ

	Lateral View	X ray – Lateral View	Dorsoplantar View	X ray – Dorsoplantar View
Signs of STJ pronation	Closed sinus tarsi Anterior portion of the lateral process of talus contacts with floor of the sinus Increased overlapping between talar head and anterior process of the calcaneus Anterior STJ not clearly appreciated Fibula placed near the tibial midline		Increased divergence of the talo-calcaneal angle A large "V" may be drawn between the anterior processes of talus and calcaneus	
Representation of pronation and supination in weight-bearing x-rays	Lateral view		Dorsoplantar view	

Signs of STJ supination	Wide open sinus tarsi	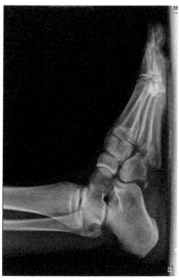		
	Decreased overlapping between talar head and anterior process of the calcaneus			
	The *canalis tarsi* is seen as a black hole between talus and calcaneus (external rotation of leg with respect to foot)			
	Orthogonal projection of STJ			
	Fibula is retropositioned with respect to tibia			
		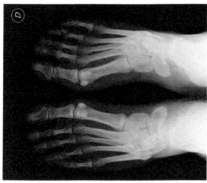		
		Decreased divergence of the talo-calcaneal angle Chopart's joint line looks like a question mark (or an "L" instead of a "V")		
		Cuboid sign (medial subluxation of the cuboid)		

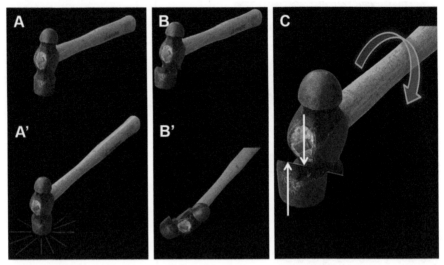

Fig. 10. Quantitative gait analysis shows that the very first ground reaction force vector does not point at the body center of mass (as it will do along the rest of the stance period), but instead is vertical, meaning each step is actually a free fall, a potentially catastrophic situation. Every initial contact is like a hammer blow of the corresponding limb, in which the head of the hammer is the heel and the handle is the tibia. If both the head and the shaft of the hammer are aligned, no turning effect will result and all of the force employed will be used for the impact (*A, A'*). But if there is a malalignment between the hammer head and its shaft, a turning effect will appear with the blow (*B, B'*). The solution is not to hold the hammer stronger but to reduce the moment arm between the action and reaction forces, such as in the "hammertomy" represented in (*C*). Straight arrows represent the pair of forces between the ground reaction force (upwards) and the force exerted through the hammer's handle (downwards; body weight & inertial forces).

An increase in the moment arm of the pair of forces (hindfoot valgus) will produce huge external (pronatory) moments that could not be balanced by internal moments. A decrease in the moment arm between the ground reaction force and the body weight will result in loss of the shock-absorbing properties of the STJ, thus increasing stress at proximal segments and joints. Distally, eversion of the calcaneus unlocks the midtarsal joint, by placing the lateral calcaneal column at the lateral side of the talar head. During closed kinetic chain STJ pronation, the calcaneus everts while the talus undergoes adduction and plantarflexion. Foot columns, medial talar and lateral calcaneal, lay one beside another at the midtarsal joint, thus allowing them to dorsiflex and providing shock absorption during the first rocker and the initial phase of the second rocker.

Second Rocker (Ankle Rocker–Plantigrade Support)

Posterior tibialis muscle decelerates the internal rotation of the tibia. It is the first of the deep posterior muscles of the leg to be activated, at around 10% of the gait cycle.[36] It contributes to achieve external rotation of the leg, which will invert the STJ, thus supinating the foot and preparing it to adopt the rigid lever anatomic arrangement (see **Fig. 5**). During the ankle rocker, STJ changes from eversion to inversion. Subtalar inversion is coupled with external rotation of the leg. Posterior tibial tendon is the best of all subtalar invertors because of both its larger moment arm and its physiologic cross-section.[28] Posterior tibial tendon pushes the medial malleolus forward, thus contributing to the external rotation of the leg, which will invert the STJ, but factors occurring above the STJ (moment of inertia of the contralateral swinging limb, the external rotators of the hip, and the biceps femoris) contribute altogether to achieve foot supination. Distally to the STJ, the windlass mechanism will contribute to foot supination once the heel is lifted at the beginning of the third rocker.[29] The soleus alone controls the forward rotation of the tibia by opposing passive ankle dorsiflexion. Gastrocnemius are not active during the second rocker; otherwise, they would tend to flex the knee while it needs to be extended to functionally lengthen the supporting limb, allowing for the opposite limb clearance.[33–35] Progressive inversion of the STJ throughout the second rocker rearranges the anatomic disposition of the foot skeleton to convert it into a rigid propulsive lever. Heel lift marks the end of the second rocker and the start of the third. By this time, the STJ is around its neutral position and will undergo additional supination throughout propulsion.

Third Rocker (Rigid Lever – Propulsion)

STJ must be inverted to allow for the Achilles-calcaneal-plantar system to act properly on the ankle joint. Loading during the third rocker consists of compressive forces between the tibia and the 3 medial metatarsals. By supinating the STJ during the second and third rockers, the foot is converted from a mobile adaptor with shock-absorbing function into a rigid lever that provides the foot with the greatest mechanical efficiency for pushing off. If the foot is pronated during the third rocker, it behaves like a bag of loose bones, leading to foot and leg fatigue secondary to overuse of muscles. A similar effect can be felt when walking on a sandy beach because of the loose properties of such a ground.

During closed kinetic chain supination, the talonavicular joint is placed over the calcaneo-cuboid joint. This arrangement is the most rigid one. The calcaneo-cuboid joint placed plantar with respect to the talonavicular joint will prevent the latter to dorsiflex. The talonavicular joint will just support axial loading or compressive stress. This joint is well prepared to cope with this kind of compressive stress during the third rocker, when the medial column adopts a vertical alignment on the ground (see **Fig. 8**). The navicular behaves as a base of support for the talar head, which lies on a tripod formed by the medial 3 rays, resembling a 3-legged stool (**Fig. 11**). A short or unstable first ray will make the navicular tilt on the medial side, leading to adduction of the talar head or medial subluxation of the talar head on the acetabulum pedis (which means foot pronation coupled to internal rotation of the leg). This deformity is referred to as lateral peritalar subluxation, because joint dislocations are usually described by the resulting deviation of the distal segment of the joint.[24]

TISSUE STRESS, DEFORMITY, PRONATORY RESERVE, AND PAIN

"Somewhat active" people walk around 9000 steps per day.[37] Cyclic loading of the musculoskeletal system represents a huge amount of stress. Bone stress is a familiar occurrence, but soft tissue stress, although often unrecognized as being a mechanical disease, is even more frequent than stress fractures. The tissue stress model allows the clinician the flexibility to adapt their evaluation and treatment procedures based on the identification of those tissues, which are swollen or injured secondary to excessive mechanical loading. Palpation, tests to stress soft tissues, the estimation of range of motion, and muscle strength should be included in the clinical examination. Posterior tibial tendon dysfunction is a common example of soft tissue stress injury, eventually ending in tendon rupture. The tendon is usually the victim of a mechanical impairment rather than its cause. Chronic rupture of the soft tissue is frequently the final stage of cyclic loading.[38]

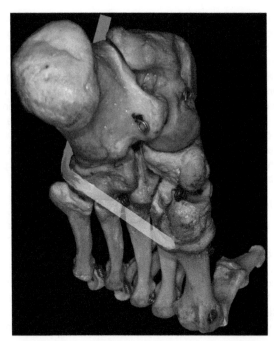

Fig. 11. During the third rocker or propulsive phase, which accounts for one-half of the stance phase, 30% of the whole cycle, the foot is vertical on the ground and the only contact area between the sole of the foot and the ground is the forefoot. The talonavicular joint lies parallel to the ground. The talus is supported by the navicular as if the latter was a three legged stool, the first three rays being the legs of the stool. During the third rocker of gait, the peroneus longus, a STJ everter in open kinetic chain conditions, stabilizes the first metatarsal against the ground by plantar flexing it and provides the STJ with an invertor stabilizing moment. It pushes the cuboid medially thus contributing to set the calcaneal foot underneath the talar foot.

Pathomechanical Syndromes of the Subtalar Joint

Specifically at the STJ, symptoms may arise as the consequence of excessive pronation or supination. There is no direct correlation between the apparent degree of deformity and the degree of pain and disability. A foot with an apparently normal alignment may present with symptoms of excessive pronation or supination. However, in most cases, those feet with medially deviation of the STJ axis will present with signs and symptoms derived from increased medial tensile stress and increased lateral compressive stress on the lateral aspect of the STJ, whereas feet with a lateral deviation of the STJ axis will suffer from increased medial compressive stress and lateral tensile stress. Increased stress may lead to pain, swelling, tissue rupture, and deformity. Pain can be explained by the stimulation of nociceptors because of increased loading. Microruptures of daily living activities may overwhelm the tissue's auto-repairing capability. Deformity becomes evident with tissue failure.

Pronatory syndromes

Symptoms and signs related to hindfoot pronation include those derived from (1) increased medial tensile soft tissue stress and/or (2) increased lateral bony compression.

1. Medial soft tissue structures include the invertor tendons (posterior tibial tendon, flexor digitorum longus, and flexor hallucis longus), the medial region of the acetabulum pedis, the spring ligament, the medial collateral ligament complex (deep tibiotalar ligament, and the superficial layer of the deltoid ligament). All these structures may show inflammatory changes in image procedures at a different degree. At the most plantar region, the plantar fascia may show the consequence of tensile stress developing plantar fibromatosis, pain (often referred to as plantar fasciitis), and even rupture. Once soft tissue damage leads to breakage of the acetabulum pedis, the talar head may protrude medially. The navicular may be abducted, causing uncovering of the talar head. The foot may be externally rotated with foot abduction, representing relative shortening of the lateral column with respect to the medial column. The skin may show keratotic lesions at the medial side of the foot. The leg is internally rotated with respect to the foot, and the capability of the posterior tibial tendon to externally rotate the leg is progressively lost. The tendon may be elongated and dysfunctional with or without evidence of rupture.

2. Lateral bony compression in the pronated STJ frequently presents with sinus tarsi pain. At the initial stages, compression of the soft tissues contained in the sinus may be painful. Finally, true direct bony impingement between the lateral process of the talus and the floor of the sinus tarsi may be the block that stops pronation. In the long-standing pronated foot, a synovial joint may develop between the lateral process of the talus and the prethalamic surface of the calcaneus. Eventually, an impingement between the fibula and the calcaneus may develop. This impingement is particularly frequent in tarsal coalition with a ball-and-socket ankle joint or in severe hindfoot valgus deformity. Symptoms in these patients may be due to the compressive stress between the lateral malleolus and the lateral surface of the calcaneus, with or without peroneal tendon impingement. Osteoarthritic changes may develop at the calcaneo-cuboid joint. Another location of bone stress related to increased compression in the pronated foot is the fibula. Stress fractures of the distal fibula present in cases of peritalar collapse.

The pronatory reserve is the capability to pronate from the most pronated position of the STJ during gait.[39] It has been suggested that lack of additional pronation due to a stop by the posterior tibial tendon, the plantar aponeurosis, and the sinus tarsi will be painful, whereas a foot with pronated alignment but additional pronatory motion will not be painful.[40] On one hand, it is evident by the authors' clinical experience that a number of flat feet will never develop any pain or disability. On the other hand, apparently normally aligned feet may present with a pronatory syndrome. For instance, in a patient with genu varum, the inclination of the tibia with respect to the ground may force the STJ into maximal pronation, producing a pronatory syndrome despite foot alignment that may resemble varus.

Supinatory syndromes
Symptoms and signs related to hindfoot supination include those derived from (1) increased lateral tensile soft tissue stress and/or (2) increased medial bony compression.

As a rule, a pronated foot is not necessarily pathologic, but a supinated foot usually is, with or without an underlying neurologic disease.

1. Symptoms of increased tensile stress at the lateral side of the STJ include lateral ankle instability and pain at the peroneal tendons. During visual gait analysis, extensor overrecruitment may be observed. Persistent activity of the long extensor tendons during the second rocker may appear as a consequence of ankle equinus

or hindfoot varus. Ankle equinus may be excessive for a normal tibialis anterior tendon to cope with increased plantar flexor moments. However, in this setting, the increase in the strength and/or timing in the action of the long extensors during the swing phase and the first and second rockers of gait is a compensatory mechanism to cope with an increased supinatory moment of the STJ. Hindfoot varus may exceed the capability of the peroneus brevis to balance the foot during the stance. When the calcaneal tuberosity lies medial to the axis of the tibia, external moments at the STJ after the initial contact will be supinatory, which will stress the peroneus brevis and may undergo degenerative tendinopathy and eventually rupture. The long extensor tendons of the toes provide the STJ with an extrapronatory moment in an attempt to balance the foot during the swing phase and the first 2 rockers.

2. Increased compression at the medial side of the STJ often is suffered proximally, at the tibia. Apart from stress fractures of the tibia, lack of STJ pronation after the initial contact may increase the stress on the knee joint that tries to cope with the additional shock absorption requirements. The skin may show keratosis at the lateral border of the foot, particularly at the fifth metatarsal. A keratosis strictly plantar to the first metatarsal head may develop when there is significant plantar flexion of the bone as a cause of hindfoot varus.

In both pronatory and supinatory syndromes, reducing the mechanical stress on the injured area will promote healing and restore flexibility and strength of the involved tissues.[38] Both nonoperative and operative management strategies regarding the STJ should aim to restore balance between the external and the internal moments, thus reducing tissue stress.

CORRELATION BETWEEN SUBTALAR JOINT MECHANICS AND DECISION-MAKING IN THE TREATMENT OF ITS PATHOLOGIC CONDITIONS

Understanding STJ pathomechanics provides a framework for surgical planning. It is important to identify mechanical impairment and to define what is the mechanical effect needed to change a pathologic condition. It is also important to know what the initial problem is and what the consequences are in terms of soft tissue or bony stress leading to peritalar injury. Whenever possible, one should try to operate to change pathomechanics and facilitate spontaneous repair of stressed structures.

Based on the normal and pathologic function of the foot, there will be several mechanical effects that would be advisable to achieve. By means of a surgical procedure, moment arms can be modified around the STJ. The internal forces can be increased or reduced. One can also consider operating on structures distant from the STJ itself, on the foot and leg segments. Finally, STJ motion can be limited or blocked as the appropriate mechanical effect in certain conditions.

Modification of Moment Arms

An osteotomy is an easy, effective, and reproducible way to modify moments acting on the STJ. By medially displacing the calcaneal tuberosity, the external pronatory moment acting around the STJ at heel contact can be reduced (Koutsogiannis effect). Conversely, lateral displacement osteotomies of the tuberosity will increase the external pronatory moment. The modification of the moment arm of the pair formed by ground reaction force and net body force (gravity and inertia acting on the body mass) allows the surgeon to control the net moment acting on the STJ. If the calcaneal tuberosity is placed exactly under the STJ axis, the external moment acting on the joint will be zero. Coaxial alignment of both calcaneal tuberosity and the projected body weight will eliminate the capability of the peritalar complex for shock absorption during the loading response. If the calcaneal tuberosity lies medial to the projected line of action of the body weight, the net external moment at the initial contact will be supinatory.

Single-plane retrothalamic osteotomies of the calcaneus allow the surgeon to medially or laterally displace the tuberosity (**Fig. 12**). Their effect does not depend on the distance from the osteotomy plane to the calcaneal tuberosity. Elevation and lowering of the tuberosity are additional optional effects in STJ surgery. The Dwyer effect consists of the lateralization of the tuberosity by means of an external base resection osteotomy. The closer to the tuberosity, the less the lateralizing effect provided by the procedure.

Retrothalamic lengthening of the calcaneus will increase the plantar flexor moment arm of the Achilles-calcaneus-plantar system. However, prethalamic lengthening of the calcaneus (Evans effect) will result in lateral column lengthening; the procedure is useful in cases of talar head uncovering with abduction at the midtarsal joint. The Evans effect will produce an internal rotation of the navicular, which provides the

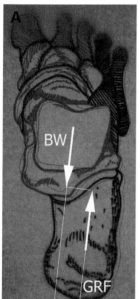
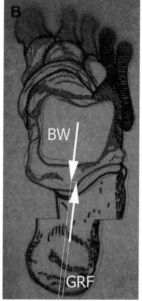
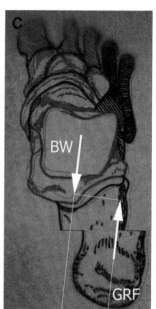

Fig. 12. In the normally aligned foot, the axis of the tibia and the axis of the calcaneus are not coincident. The axis of the calcaneal tuberosity lies slightly lateral to the projected axis of the tibia (*A*). A pair of forces is created between the ground reaction force and the body weight, which in turn generates a pronatory external moment. This is the reason why in static stance, the STJ tends to adopt a mild valgus alignment. By medially displacing the calcaneal tuberosity (*B*), the moment arm for external forces is reduced. After medial sliding of the calcaneal tuberosity (Koutsogiannis effect), the external pronatory moment is markedly reduced for a given load. Lateral sliding of the tuberosity (reversed Koutsogiannis) has the opposite effect, increasing the passive pronatory external moment (*C*). The surgeon can modify moments acting on a joint by acting on the active element or on the lever arms. It is obviously more predictable to act on the moment arms of both the external and the internal sources of force. Arrows represent force vectors BW and GRF (BW, body weight; GRF, ground reaction force). By medially displacing the calcaneal tuberosity the moment arm of the pair of forces is reduced. Conversely, by lateralizing the calcaneal tuberosity, the moment arm of the pair of forces is increased, thus increasing the external pronatory moment at the STJ after the initial contact.

STJ with an additional supinatory moment.[39] The resulting position of the first metatarsal head should be checked out because it may suffer elevation and then require additional procedures to plantarflex the first ray.

Procedures Modifying Internal Forces

These procedures can be divided into soft tissue repair and augmentation procedures and releasing procedures.

Both tendon repair and tendon transfers aim to increase internal moments acting on the force generators instead of on the lever arms. From a theoretic point of view, it is a valid way to increase internal moments. However, these procedures have some disadvantages. The transferred tendon will probably generate less force, and the firing pattern of the muscle and the new tribology of the tendon may not be good enough to provide the STJ with the desired force. It should be noted that if a previously healthy tendon has failed and undergone chronic rupture as a consequence of increased soft tissue stress, it is unlikely that, by simply replacing it with another tendon, function will be restored. All of these reasons favor operations on lever arms rather than on internal force generators in patients with primary mechanical STJ pathologic condition. Currently, the authors do not repair any ruptured posterior tibial tendon in the pronatory syndromes or the peroneus brevis in the STJ supinatory syndromes. They try to provide the STJ with adequate balance, which usually means operating on different and distant structures to reduce external moments.

The second group of procedures to modify force generation includes soft tissue release of contracture or congenitally short soft tissue. It is well known the harmful effect that a simple anatomic variant, such as the length ratio between the tibia and the triceps, may produce on the STJ.[24,41,42] In normal conditions, the Achilles tendon exerts a supinatory moment on the STJ. Ankle equinus is a restraint to passive dorsiflexion of the ankle joint. Under such circumstances, particularly if the ankle block takes place at around 90°, STJ pronation may occur as a compensatory mechanism to provide for the additional foot dorsiflexion necessary to accomplish the second rocker. It is interesting to point out that severe equinus will affect mostly the forefoot. However, it is mild equinus (that around the neutral position) with increased resistance to passive foot dorsiflexion from neutral that may affect both the plantar fascia and the integrity of the plantar vault, by means of increased pronation as a compensatory mechanism to achieve the required foot/leg dorsiflexion at the end of the second rocker. In the particular case of the STJ, selective or total triceps lengthening are common procedures in the management of the pronated foot.

Modification of the Leg and Foot Segments

Because the STJ may be painful as a result of mechanical impairments produced at a distance from the hindfoot itself, the surgeon must be aware to identify them to avoid operating on the victim rather than on the culprit. For instance, knee malalignment or instability may generate STJ pathologic condition. Some cases of knee varus may not present with knee pain but with a pronatory syndrome instead. This syndrome is particularly frequent in patients with marked medial inclination of the tibia, whose STJ are maximally pronated to allow for plantigrade foot contact on the ground. The foot may show a normal or even supinated alignment, but the medial soft tissues or the sinus tarsi suffer the consequence of increased pronatory stress. A ruptured posterior tibial tendon may in this case need a proximal tibial valgus osteotomy. Some patients with anterior cruciate ligament instability may present with a pronatory syndrome as well. Both pronatory and supinatory syndromes may appear in the case of knee valgus deformity.

At the distal segment, forefoot intrinsic malalignment can affect the STJ. It is important to assess the relative position of the forefoot with respect to the hindfoot. Primary plantarflexion of the first metatarsal (forefoot valgus) may produce a supinating moment at the STJ. The Coleman block test is a useful clinical test to address whether STJ varus may be the consequence of the distal impairment. Also, STJ pronation may increase dorsiflexing moments at the medial forefoot, resulting in first metatarsal elevation. Whenever planning any surgical procedure to restore STJ function or alignment, interventions on the midfoot and the forefoot should be considered as combined procedures if needed.

Procedures Reducing or Blocking Subtalar Joint Motion

An arthroereisis is a procedure designed to limit joint motion to a certain range. In the particular case of the STJ, arthroereisis limiting hindfoot pronation has been widely used, particularly among European surgeons. Because the supinated STJ presents with a wide open sinus tarsi, blocking the cavity with an implant or placing a screw at the posterior calcaneal facet will prevent the lateral process of the talus from advancing toward the prethalamic surface or floor of the sinus tarsi. Because the sinus tarsi remains opened, the STJ will be inverted. Temporary correction of valgus deformity in children may provide for joint remodeling, thus allowing for permanent correction after implant removal. In the adult, permanent corrections have been described as well, although additional bony or soft tissue procedures are usually combined with the arthroereisis. When dealing with flexible pronatory syndromes (stage 2 flatfoot deformity),[43] the authors prefer not to limit STJ motion.

Fusion of the STJ may be indicated to eliminate pain in certain arthritic STJ or to provide stability in cases of deficient motor control. Stage 3 flatfoot deformity may need STJ fusion with or without additional local joint fusions. In the case of mechanical impairments, the authors may decide whether fusion is needed on the basis of the clinical examination: if there is painless STJ motion, the authors try to preserve it no matter what the radiological appearance of the STJ. If there is no passive STJ motion or the remaining motion is painful in non-weight-bearing conditions, the authors prefer to fuse the STJ no matter if it is apparently healthy in image studies. When forefoot malalignment results following STJ fusion, the midtarsal joint is likely to be included in the procedure. Local joint pain is a valid criterion for triple arthrodesis. In the management of cavovarus deformity, triple arthrodesis is used more frequently, both for motor control in the neurologic patient and for the correction of a severely supinated foot.

In the authors' practice, there is an additional indication for STJ fusion, no matter the previous status of the joint itself: in the case of an ankle fusion, they routinely fuse the STJ as well, making sure it remains in the pronated position. Loss of the tibiotalar joint motion is a catastrophic impairment from the mechanical point of view. Once the ankle joint motion is lost, the main mechanical issue of the patient is loss of the second rocker. Loss of the second rocker may be partially compensated by the midtarsal joint but not by the STJ.[44] By fusing the STJ in valgus at the time of tibiotalar fusion, the midtarsal joint is provided with the maximum passive dorsiflexion possible, because both columns of the foot are displayed one beside the other. In the setting of a tibiotalar arthrodesis, if the STJ is left unfused, it will be blocked in varus in the midterm, thus resulting in decreased foot dorsiflexion.[44] As a general rule, a little STJ varus is too much varus. However, in the case of STJ fusion, the slightest varus is unacceptable. When operating on severe long-term valgus deformities, overcorrection should be especially avoided because pain may be disabling despite improvement of both radiographs and clinical appearance of the foot. The authors prefer to use arthrodesis in flatfeet as stabilizers rather than corrective procedures.

REFERENCES

1. Viladot A, Lorenzo JC, Salazar J, et al. The subtalar joint. Embryology and morphology. Foot Ankle Int 1984;5(2):54–66.
2. Martinez-Cuadrado G. Formación y desarrollo de la arteria del seno del tarso en embriones y fetos humanos. Ph.D. Thesis, Facultad de Medicina, Universidad de Madrid, 1965.
3. Palma de L, Santucci A, Ventura A, et al. Anatomy and embryology of the talocalcaneal joint. Foot Ankle Surg 2003;9(1):7–18.
4. Basmajian JV. Surface anatomy: an instructional manual. Baltimore (MD): Williams & Wilkins; 1983.
5. Testut L, Latarjet A. Tratado de anatomia humana. Barcelona (Spain): Salvat; 1988.
6. Von Volkmann R. Ein ligamentum "neglectum" pedís (Ligamenta calcaneonaviculare mediodorsale seu sustentaculonaviculare). Verh Anat Ges 1970;64:483–90 [in German].
7. Schmidt HM. Shape and fixation of band systems in human sinus and canalis tarsi. Acta Anat 1978;102:184.
8. Cahill DR. The anatomy and function of the contents of the human tarsal sinus and canal. Anat Rec 1965;153(1):1–17.
9. Harper MC. The lateral ligamentous support of the subtalar joint. Foot Ankle 1991; 11(6):354–8.
10. Jones FW. The talocalcaneal articulation. Lancet 1944;22:241–2.
11. Stagni R, Leardini A, O'Connor JJ, et al. Role of passive structures in the mobility and stability of the human subtalar joint: a literature review. Foot Ankle Int 2003; 24(5):402–9.
12. Stephens MM, Sammarco GJ. The stabilizing role of the lateral ligament complex around the ankle and subtalar joints. Foot Ankle 1992;13(3):130–6.
13. Smith JW. The ligamentous structures in the canalis and sinus tarsi. J Anat 1958; 92:612–20.
14. Sanz TA. Estudio anatómico y funcional de la articulación subastragalina. Diseño de una prótesis para la articulación subastragalina posterior. Ph.D. Thesis, Facultad de Medicina, Universidad de Extremadura, 1992.
15. Hicks JH. The mechanics of the foot. I. The joints. J Anat 1953;87:345–57.
16. Henke W. Handbuch der Anatomie und Mechanik der Gelenke. Heidelberg (Germany): CF Wintersche Verlashandlung; 1863. Available at: http://www.mdz-nbn-resolving.de/urn/resolver.pl?urn=urn:nbn:de:bvb:12-bsb10368491-1.
17. Seibel M. Foot function: a programmed text. Baltimore (MD): Williams & Wilkins; 1988.
18. Kapandji IA. Physiologie articulaire. Fascicule II. Paris (France): Librairie Maloine SA; 1970.
19. Manter JT. Movements of the subtalar and transverse tarsal joints. Anat Rec 1941; 46(3):469–81.
20. Isman RE, Inman VT. Anthropometric studies of the human foot and ankle. Bull Prosthet Res 1969;10:97–129.
21. Van Langelaan EJ. A kinematic analysis of the tarsal joints: an x-ray photogrammetric study. Acta Orthop Scand 1983;54(Suppl):135–229.

22. Bonnel F, Faure P, Nicoleau F, et al. L'articulation sous-talienne. In: Herisson C, Borderie P, Simon L, editors. La Pathologie de L'Articulation Sous-Talienne. Paris (France): Masson; 1994. p. 1–8.

23. Núñez-Samper M, Llanos-Alcázar LF. Exploración clínica y complementaria. In: Núñez-Samper M, Llanos-Alcázar LF, editors. Biomecánica, medicina y cirugía del pie. 2nd edition. Barcelona (Spain): Masson; 2007. p. 103–10.

24. Hansen ST. Functional reconstruction of the foot and ankle. Philadelphia: Lippincott Williams & Wilkins; 2000.

25. Lundberg A, Svensson OK, Bylund C, et al. Kinematics of the ankle/foot complex. Part 2: pronation and supination. Foot Ankle Int 1989;9(5):248–53.

26. Lundberg A, Svensson OK. The axes of rotation of the talocalcaneal and talonavicular joints. Foot 1993;3:65–70.

27. Gellman H, Lenihan M, Halikis N, et al. Selective tarsal arthrodesis: an in vitro analysis of the effect on foot motion. Foot Ankle Int 1987;8(3):127–33.

28. Silver RL, de la Garza J, Rang M. They myth of muscle balance. J Bone Joint Surg Br 1985;67(3):432–7.

29. Kirby KA. Methods for determination of positional variations in the subtalar joint axis. J Am Podiatr Med Assoc 1987;77(5):228–34.

30. Kirby KA. Subtalar joint axis location and rotational equilibrium theory of foot function. J Am Podiatr Med Assoc 2001;91:465–87.

31. Roukis TS, Kirby KA. A simple intraoperative technique to accurately align the rearfoot complex. J Am Podiatr Med Assoc 2005;95(5):505–7.

32. Viladot A. Quince lecciones sobre patología del pie. Barcelona (Spain): Toray; 1989.

33. Perry J, Schoneberger B. Gait analysis: normal and pathological function. Thorofare (NJ): Slack Inc; 1992.

34. Gage JR, DeLuca PA, Renshaw TS. Gait analysis: principles and applications. J Bone Joint Surg Am 1995;77(10):1607–23.

35. Kirtley C. Clinical gait analysis. Theory and practice. Oxford (United Kingdom): Churchill-Livingstone, Elsevier; 2006.

36. Sutherland DH. An electromyographic study of the plantar flexors of the ankle in normal walking on the level. J Bone Joint Surg Am 1966;48A(1):66–71.

37. Tudor-Locke C, Bassett DR Jr. How many steps/day are enough? Preliminary pedometer indices for public health. Sports Med 2004;34(1):1–8.

38. McPoil TG, Hunt GC. Evaluation and management of foot and ankle disorders: present problems and future directions. J Orthop Sports Phys Ther 1995;21(6): 381–8.

39. Pascual-Huerta J, Ropa-Moreno JM, Kirby KA. Static response of maximally pronated and nonmaximally pronated feet to frontal plane wedging of foot orthoses. J Am Podiatr Med Assoc 2009;99:13–9.

40. Fuller E. Center of pressure and its theoretical relationship to foot pathology. J Am Podiatr Med Assoc 1999;89(6):278–91.

41. De Doncker E, Kowalski C. Cinesiologie et reeducation du pied. Paris (France): Masson; 1979.

42. Barouk LS, Barouk P. Gastrocnemius tightness. From anatomy to treatment. Montpellier (France): Sauramps; 2012.

43. Bluman EM, Title CI, Myerson MS, et al. Posterior tibial tendon rupture: a refined classification system. Foot Ankle Clin 2007;8(3):637–45.

44. Viladot Pericé A, Dalmau A. Tratamiento de las secuelas postraumáticas del miembro inferior. Fundación Mapfre. Temas Medicina 1988;30:535–43.

Imaging of the Subtalar Joint

Robert Lopez-Ben, MD[a,b]

KEYWORDS

• Ankle • Hindfoot • Radiography • MRI • Computed tomography • Ultrasound

KEY POINTS

- Although the complex anatomy of the subtalar joint can be delineated with oblique radiographic views, it is better represented with CT or MRI.
- The anterior and posterior subtalar joint do not typically communicate during arthrography.
- MRI improves detection of subtalar coalition and CT is critical in assessing subtalar involvement with calcaneal and talar fractures.

Imaging of the subtalar joint can be challenging because of its complex planar anatomy and the breadth of pathology that can involve this joint. Radiography remains the initial mode of imaging but frequently, cross-sectional imaging is needed to better fully appreciate the joint anatomy and improve the sensitivity and the specificity of detection of pathology involving the subtalar joint. Arthrography of the joint is rarely used as a strict diagnostic imaging modality in current clinical practice but is commonly used before the intra-articular injection of local anesthetic and corticosteroid.

OSSEOUS ANATOMY

The subtalar joint is the articulation between the calcaneus and talus. It is typically divided into three articulating facets of the superior calcaneus: (1) anterior, (2) middle, and (3) posterior. The anterior joint is variably present and is the smallest component of the subtalar joint.[1] The anterior facet articulates with the head of the talus. It lies anterior and slightly lateral to the middle facet. The middle facet is centered at the sustentaculum tali. The middle facet portion of the joint can communicate with the talonavicular joint.[2] Both the anterior and middle facets are concave.

The posterior facet of the subtalar joint is the largest. It articulates the undersurface of the talar body with the calcaneus. It is slightly convex. The posterior facet is separated from the anterior and middle facet by the nonosseous sinus tarsi. The sinus tarsi

The Author has nothing to disclose.
[a] Department of Radiology, University of North Carolina School of Medicine at Charlotte, NC 27516, USA; [b] Charlotte Radiology, 1701 East Boulevard, Charlotte, NC 28203, USA
E-mail address: bobrlopez@gmail.com

has the shape of a cone.[3] The base of the cone is widest at its lateral margin and narrows as it courses medially. The most medial portion of the sinus tarsi is also referred to as the tarsal canal.[4]

The planes of the middle and posterior facets are parallel and inclined 45 degrees anteriorly with respect to the long axis of the calcaneus.[5] In relation to the sole of the foot, the anterior portions of these facets are angled inferiorly between 25 and 40 degrees.[6]

Some common anatomic variations in this area of the subtalar joint include an absent anterior facet or a joint anterior and middle facet. There is an association with an increased incidence of degenerative arthritis in patients that do not have a separate anterior and middle facet, perhaps caused by increased biomechanical subtalar joint stability when both the anterior and middle facets are present.[7] Another recognized anatomic variant is that the posterior margin of the sustentaculum tali can extend medially with an accessory facet articulating with the posteromedial talar process.[8]

RADIOGRAPHY

An understanding of the anatomy of the subtalar joint is helpful to appreciate the several overlapping structures that on standard lateral radiographic projection can decrease the sensitivity of detection of pathology. Because of the previously mentioned obliquity of the joint surfaces and the superimposition of these complex three-dimensional osseous components of the subtalar joint on a two-dimensional radiograph, a standard anterior to posterior view of the foot or ankle fails to visualize the joint effectively. Lateral radiographs of the foot and ankle depict some overlap between the posterior and middle facets. The lateral process of the talus can usually be identified and can help identify the anterior margin of the posterior facet on a lateral view (**Fig. 1**).[9] Oblique radiographic projections can be performed to improve the delineation of the joint surfaces.

An axial calcaneal projection, also named a Harris-Beath view, can demonstrate the middle and posterior facets of the subtalar joint, with a tangential projection of the sustentaculum tali and posterior calcaneal body (**Fig. 2**). The central radiographic beam is

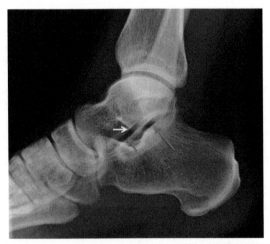

Fig. 1. Lateral radiograph of the foot and ankle. *Yellow arrow* denotes lateral talar body process. *Long blue arrow* shows posterior facet and *short blue arrow* shows middle facet of the subtalar joint. Note the parallel orientation of the facets and their inferior anterior angulation with respect to the calcaneal body long axis.

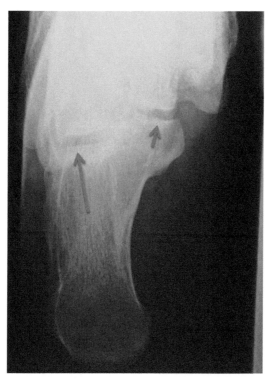

Fig. 2. Harris view of the calcaneus. *Long arrow* shows posterior facet and *short arrow* shows middle facet of the subtalar joint.

centered in the posterior facet of the joint and angled up to 45 degrees posteriorly toward the midline of the heel.

Broden view has been used to view the posterior facet in a lateral projection. The patient is supine with the leg internally rotated 30 to 45 degrees. The center beam is placed in the lateral malleolus. The x-ray tube is then angled sequentially in 10-degree increments from 10 to 40 degrees cephalad (**Fig. 3**).

A lateral oblique axial projection can also image the posterior facet of the joint in profile. The foot is dorsiflexed and slightly everted. The leg is laterally rotated 60 degrees, flexing the knee with the foot rested on a 30-degree wedge. The tube is then tilted 10-degrees cephalad, with the center beam located 1 inch below the medial malleolus.[10]

Less commonly performed, a medial oblique axial view can demonstrate the middle facet. The foot is dorsiflexed and inverted. The leg is rotated medially 60 degrees and the foot again rested on a 30-degree wedge. The tube is directed axially, tilted 10 degrees toward the head and centered 1 inch below and 1 inch anterior to the lateral malleolus (**Fig. 4**).[10]

COMPUTED TOMOGRAPHY AND MRI

Multidetector computed tomography (CT) can acquire axial images helically through the joint, with multplanar reformations reconstructed of an isotropic data set. Two-dimensional reformations in the coronal and sagittal planes can be reconstructed with different obliquities.

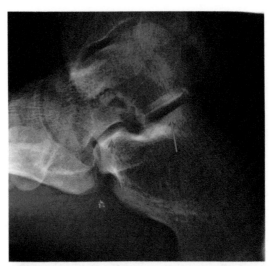

Fig. 3. Lateral oblique projection with 30 degrees of central radiographic beam angulation cephalad showing separation of the posterior and middle facets. *Long arrow* shows posterior facet and *short arrow* shows middle facet of the subtalar joint.

At our institution, using a 16-channel multidetector CT scanner, the hindfoot is imaged with 0.625-mm collimation, a pitch of 0.5625, 120 kVp, and 200 mA to create a near isotropic dataset. When imaging the subtalar joint, sagittal and coronal reformatted images are prescribed perpendicularly off the axial images of the tibiotalar joint. When imaging for calcaneal fractures, to better use the Sanders classification,

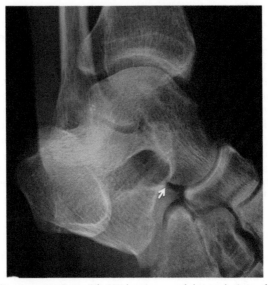

Fig. 4. Medial oblique projection with 20 degrees caudal angulation of the central beam showing the anterior facet (*arrow*).

coronal reformations are prescribed of the sagittal images perpendicular to the posterior facet as opposed to the tibiotalar joint.

Further postprocessing with a volumetric three-dimensional reconstruction can be performed in cases of complex fracture patterns to better evaluate the relationships of the comminuted fracture fragments with each other (**Fig. 5**). Also, cone beam CT and tomosynthesis are novel technologies that can allow upright weight-bearing during imaging. Evaluation of the hindfoot alignment and subtalar joint width and position during weight-bearing when compared with the standard non–weight-bearing conventional CT has shown significant differences and could prove helpful in the evaluation of the planovalgus foot or dynamic subfibular impingement (**Fig. 6**).[11]

MRI of the hindfoot is routinely performed to evaluate subtalar joint pathology. As with CT, multiplanar imaging allows for a better appreciation of the complex anatomy of this joint. The inherent increased soft tissue contrast of MRI when compared with CT allows for depiction of any associated hindfoot tendon and ligament pathology. Increased T2 and decreased T1 signal within the marrow (ie, marrow edema) of the talus and calcaneus can help identify marrow contusions and microtrabecular fractures and reactive trabecular changes from altered biomechanics.[12] **Table 1** shows the routine sequences and imaging parameters for MRI of the ankle and hindfoot at our institution. A coronal T1 series can be helpful and may be added to the previously mentioned sequences when evaluating for tarsal coalition.

Ligamentous Anatomy

Because of its soft tissue contrast resolution, MRI is also able to depict the ligamentous anatomy of the joint. Apart from the subtalar joint capsule, the extracapsular ligament support of this joint includes the calcaneofibular ligament laterally, the superficial deltoid ligament medially, and the ligaments of the sinus tarsi. The sinus

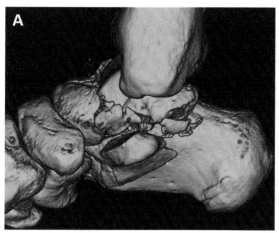
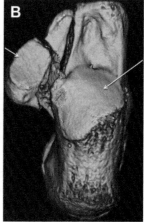

Fig. 5. (*A*) Three-dimensional reformation of hindfoot CT in a patient with complex talar neck and body fracture with calcaneal extension through the subtalar joint. (*B*) Same three-dimensional CT reformation after postprocessing removal of the talus allowing for isolated depiction of the calcaneus. The image is oriented to show the superior surface of the calcaneus. Note the longitudinal fracture line through the sustentaculum tali displacing the middle facet of the subtalar joint (*short arrow*) with relative sparing of the posterior facet (*long arrow*).

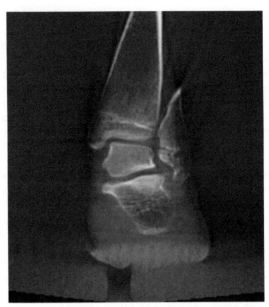

Fig. 6. Weight-bearing coronal tomographic view showing preservation of the posterior facet subtalar joint space and possible mild hindfoot valgus.

tarsi contains fat, with nerves, vessels, and ligaments coursing within it. These sinus tarsi ligaments can help limit hindfoot inversion. These ligaments include, from lateral to medial, the inferior extensor retinaculum, the cervical ligament, and the talocalcaneal interosseus ligament. The latter may have a variable appearance with a band-type most prevalent in a cadaveric study, with fan-type and multifasciular ligament morphology also identified.[13]

The posterior facet of the subtalar joint has thickening of the joint capsule that lends ligamentous support to the joint. Some of the more defined intracapsular ligaments are the posterior and lateral talocalcaneal and the anterior capsular ligaments that reinforce the joint capsule.

The subtalar joint can also have common anatomic variations in its ligamentous contents. The medial talocalcaneal ligament attaches from the posterior aspect of the medial talar process to the sustentaculum. This ligament can be seen on magnetic resonance studies in approximately 2% of cases **(Fig. 7)**.[14] Because of this location the ligament can be confused with a fibrous tarsal collation. Similarly, there can be

Table 1
MRI of subtalar joint/hindfoot (1.5 T, Magnetom Aera, Siemens Healthcare)

Sequence	FOV	Matrix	NEX	Thick/Gap (mm)	TR (millisecond)	TE (millisecond)	TF
Sag T1	15	256 × 256	2	3/0.6	500	15	NA
Sag STIR	15	256 × 212	1	3/0.6	4000	29	8
Ax PD FSE FS	14	320 × 240	2	3/0.6	2000	49	9
Cor PD FSE FS	14	320 × 240	3	3/0.6	2000	49	10

Abbreviations: Ax, axial; Cor, coronal; FS, fat suppression; FOV, field of view; FSE, fast spin echo; NEX, number of excitations; PD, proton density; Sag, sagittal; TF, turbo factor.

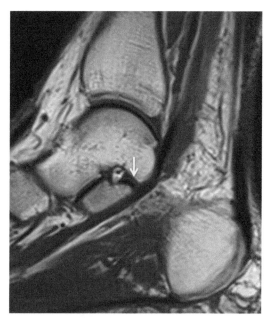

Fig. 7. Sagittal T1-weighted MRI. *Arrow* shows typical location of medial talocalcaneal capsular ligament from posteromedial talar process to the sustentaculum tali. Note the adjacent flexor hallucis longus tendon coursing inferior to the sustenaculum.

a thickening of the anterior capsular ligament that could be confused with an extra-articular fibrous coalition (**Fig. 8**).[14] However, in the setting of coalition the opposing bony surfaces are deformed and irregular in contour. Smooth bony contours and margins at the attachments of these variable ligaments can help differentiate these ligamentous variations from coalition.

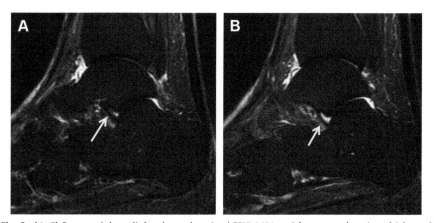

Fig. 8. (*A, B*) Sequential medial to lateral sagittal STIR MRIs, with *arrows* showing thickened anterior capsule of the posterior subtalar joint in this patient with a small amount of subtalar joint fluid.

Subtalar Joint Arthrography

The talocalcaneal joint can be divided into two separate synovial lined cavities: the anterior subtalar joint (also referred to as the talocalcaneonavicular joint), and the posterior subtalar joint (between the posterior talar facet of the calcaneus and the posterior calcaneal facet of the talus, sometimes confusingly referred to in the arthrography literature simply as the subtalar joint).[2] These two joints (anterior and posterior talocalcaneal or subtalar joints) are separated by the tarsal sinus and canal and do not normally communicate. The inferior medial capsule of the anterior subtalar joint is bordered by the plantar calcaneonavicular or spring ligament.

The anterior subtalar joint (also referred to as the talocalcaneonavicular joint) usually communicates directly with the talonavicular joint space. It does not normally communicate with the naviculocuneiform joint space (**Fig. 9**). The posterior subtalar joint space can communicate with the tibiotalar joint space of the ankle in up to 20% of some arthrography series.[2,15] This communication is usually between the posterior recesses of both joints.[16] More uncommonly, there can be communication with the common peroneal tendon sheath and/or the flexor hallucis longus tendon sheath.[17]

Given the technical advances in cross-sectional imaging for the diagnosis of subtalar joint pathology and delineation of its anatomy, arthrography of the subtalar joint is more frequently used clinically during the fluoroscopic intra-articular injection of local anesthetic and corticosteroid. An anterolateral approach to the posterior facet is technically easier to perform in most patients with less incidence of adjacent tendon sheath puncture, or in the case of the posteromedial approach, unwanted tarsal tunnel neurovascular injury.[18] In the anterolateral approach the subtalar joint is positioned in slight inversion and the needle is usually positioned anterior or superior to the adjacent peroneal tendons (**Fig. 10**). A posterolateral approach can be performed with the ankle in slight dorsiflexion and needle placement directed toward the posterior-superior joint recess. The approach can also be effective when targeting the os trigonum for injection (**Fig. 11**).

Perhaps because of its complex anatomy, fluoroscopic-guided injections of the subtalar joint have been shown to be more efficacious in pain relief than non–imaging-guided injections using clinical landmarks.[19] However, even with experienced operators, extra-articular injections can be seen in 15% of patients, usually because of

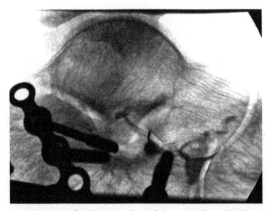

Fig. 9. Spot fluoroscopy image of arthrography of the anterior subtalar joint using a medial approach. Care must be taken with this approach to avoid the medial neurovascular structures within the tarsal tunnel. This patient had prior calcaneal fracture with lateral reconstruction plate and screws. Contrast does not communicate with the posterior facet.

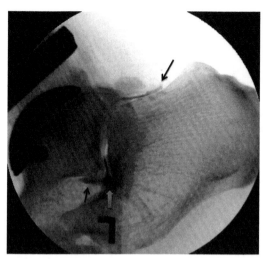

Fig. 10. Patient with prior total ankle arthroplasty with recurring ankle pain referred for injection of local anesthetic and corticosteroid within the posterior subtalar joint. Spot fluoroscopy image shows 25-gauge needle (*blue arrow*) placed via anterolateral approach. Initial contrast administration to document intra-articular location shows filling of the anterior and posterior joint recesses (*black arrows*). Note incidental os trigonum.

severe joint space narrowing and bridging osteophytes from underlying degenerative joint pathology or prior traumatic deformity.[18] Alternative imaging-guided approaches, such as CT, allow direct visualization of the joint space and overlying structures but this imaging modality is not as commonly used because of its possible increased radiation exposure and more limited availability in many clinical settings (**Fig. 12**). More recently, ultrasound guidance has been proposed as a viable alternative for imaging guidance to the subtalar joint with 100% efficacy of intra-articular access noted in a small cadaveric series using anterolateral, posteromedial, and posterolateral approaches.[20]

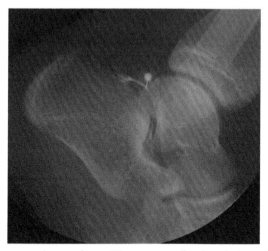

Fig. 11. Spot fluoroscopy image shows 25-gauge needle placed via posterior and lateral approach at junction of os trigonum and posterior joint recess. Initial contrast administration to document intra-articular location shows filling of posterior subtalar joint.

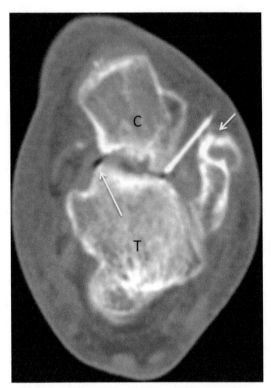

Fig. 12. Patient with severe posttraumatic deformity of the posterior subtalar joint resulting in prior fluoroscopic failure of intra-articular injection. CT fluoroscopy image of injection of the posterior subtalar joint with the patient prone. A 25-gauge needle has been inserted posterior to the peroneal tendons, which have contrast within the common peroneal tendon sheath (*short arrow*) from prior unsuccessful fluoroscopic injection attempt. Small amount of air documents intra-articular location (*long arrow*). C, calcaneus; T, talus. (*Courtesy of* Brian Howard, MD, Charlotte, NC.)

Imaging of Talocalcaneal Coalition

Tarsal coalition is an abnormal bridging of two bones that are normally separated by an articulation. It is usually caused by an abnormal developmental failure of mesenchymal differentiation and segmentation. It can be a synostosis that is composed of fibrous, cartilaginous, or osseous tissues. The imaging differentiation between cartilaginous and fibrous coalition cannot be directly visualized with CT but can be suggested by MRI, which can show the bridging fibrous tissue as decreased signal intensity on all pulse sequences.[14]

Talocalcaneal coalitions can be intra-articular or extra-articular. Intra-articular talocalcaneal coalitions usually involve the middle facet.[21] Intra-articular coalitions can occur much less frequently in the posterior facets and usually partially involve the posterior-medial joint surface.[22] There may be bony overgrowth of the posterior medial aspect of the posterior subtalar joint into the tarsal tunnel with potential impingement of the neurovascular structures coursing within it, and superior overgrowth of the posterior calcaneal facet with a humpback-type deformity.[23] Intra-articular coalitions of the anterior facet are rarely isolated, and when they occur, also typically involve the adjacent middle facet.[21] Extra-articular coalitions usually involve the posterior margin of the sustentaculum tali and the adjacent posterior margin of the medial talar process.[14,24]

Osseous intra-articular coalitions are more apparent on radiographs or imaging because of the conspicuity of the bridging bone on CT or MRI. They usually ossify between the ages of 12 and 16 as the patient becomes skeletally mature and thus become easier to detect on radiography and imaging.[25] Radiographs may show inability to detect the middle subtalar joint, and secondary signs, such as talar beaking (**Fig. 13**).[9,26] The latter is believed to be caused by traction enthesophytes at the site of the dorsal talonavicular joint capsule attachment from the abnormal motion of the middle talocalcaneal region. Talar beaking is not specific to talocalcaneal coaltion.[27] The C-sign is present when the cortical outlines of the broadened sustentaculum tali and the talar dome form a continuous C-shaped line on the lateral radiographic view (**Fig. 14**). The C-sign, although very suggestive of a middle facet coalition, can also be seen in the setting of underlying hindfoot valgus.[28] On weight-bearing lateral views of the hindfoot, the middle facet can commonly be visualized separate from the posterior facet on normal individuals. The absence of visualization of this middle facet on weight-bearing lateral views has been shown to have a 90% accuracy rate for the diagnosis of coalition in a surgically proved cohort.[9] Another radiographic sign of a subtalar coalition can be an abnormally rounded talar dome and medial and lateral gutters of the tibiotalar joint on the anterior-posterior radiograph that has been termed as a "ball and socket" ankle joint (**Fig. 15**).

Fibrous and cartilaginous coalitions may be more difficult to directly discern on CT imaging. The diagnosis can be made by identifying secondary signs, such as deformities of the osseous contours of the opposing bone surfaces. The middle facet of the subtalar joint can show inferior down sloping of its medial surfaces and the sustentaculum has a broadened articular transverse width.[29] Subchondral cystic changes in the calcaneus and talus from abnormal loading stresses in the joint can help identify underlying cartilaginous coalitions in adult patients. MRI demonstrates marrow edema at the opposing bony margins of fibrous and cartilaginous coalitions that can aid in

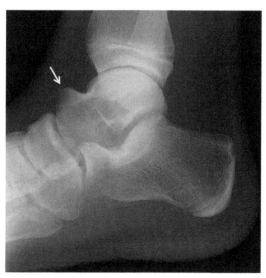

Fig. 13. Lateral radiograph of the hindfoot demonstrating talar beak (*arrow*) in a patient with surgically proved subtalar coalition.

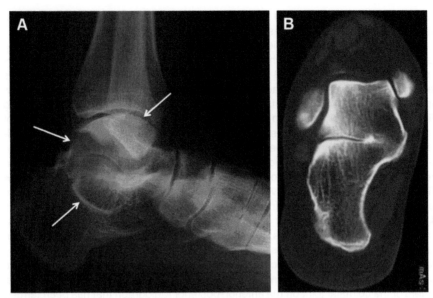

Fig. 14. (*A*) Lateral radiograph of the hindfoot shows a "C" sign (*arrows*) in this patient with osseous subtalar coalition. The apparent C-shaped line is formed by the cortical contours of the talar dome, body, and broadened sustentaculum tali. (*B*) Coronal CT of same patient showing mature osseous bridging between talus and medial facet of the subtalar joint.

their detection (**Fig. 16**).[12] Although not routinely used for diagnosis of subtalar coalition, ultrasound when used to evaluate medial ankle pain can sometimes suggest this diagnosis. A recent retrospective series of 12 patients demonstrated the ultrasound findings of subtalar coalition as a reduced joint space and irregular cortical outline when scanning the tarsal tunnel at the level of the sustentaculum tali.[30]

Imaging of Subtalar Joint Pathology

The most common indication for subtalar joint imaging is in the setting of trauma. Calcaneal fractures are the most common tarsal bone fracture. The complex anatomy of the hindfoot can limit the interpretation of radiographs for the detection of fracture and determination of their extent. Multidetector CT is the imaging examination of choice in the detection of radiographically occult fractures and in assessment of the degree of comminution and subtalar joint involvement.

Calcaneal fractures commonly involve the subtalar joint and the extent of comminution at the subtalar joint can be used for classification of these fractures. After an axial load, the primary fracture line is in the sagittal plane oriented anteromedial to posterolateral through the calcaneal body and posterior facet. The position of this fracture line in relationship to the posterior facet of the subtalar joint depends on the varus or valgus relative position of the hindfoot at the time of trauma.[31] This sagittal shear fracture splits the calcaneus into a sustentacular and a tuberosity fragment. A secondary transverse compression fracture line in the coronal plane can split the sustentacular fragment and the medial facet of the subtalar joint.

Radiographic imaging is critical in assessing if these fractures are primarily extra-articular or intra-articular in relationship to the subtalar joint, and can also estimate the degree of loss of calcaneal height by measuring Bohler angle (normally 20–40 degrees), which is formed by the intersection of a line from the most superior portion

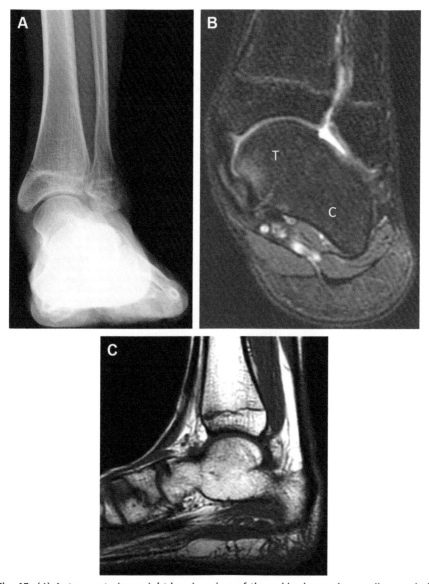

Fig. 15. (*A*) Anteroposterior weight-bearing view of the ankle shows abnormally rounded talar dome ("ball and socket joint"). (*B, C*) MRI of the same patient. (*B*) Coronal STIR imaging showing the marked osseous bridging of the subtalar joint and hindfoot valgus. (*C*) Sagittal T1-weighted image shows same findings with absence of a subtalar joint caused by bone bridge. C, calcaneus; T, talus.

of the tuberosity to the posterior margin of the posterior facet of the subtalar joint and another line from the latter position to the anterior-superior calcaneal process (**Fig. 17**).

CT is critical to assess intra-articular fractures for measurement/extent of joint depression, and comminution/incongruity of the posterior facet. CT can detect more fractures than radiography.[32] A recent study comparing Broden view with CT

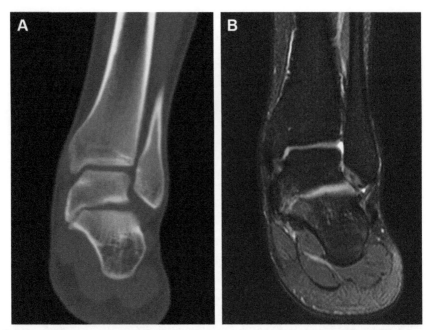

Fig. 16. Cartilaginous coalition of the medial facet. (*A*) Coronal reformatted CT image shows abnormal medial downsloping of the medial facet subtalar joint with subchondral sclerosis. (*B*) Coronal STIR MRI in the same patient showing marrow edema of the apposing articular surfaces caused by abnormal biomechanical stress.

in the assessment of intra-articular calcaneal fractures showed that the main fracture line as detected on Broden view was positioned 22% more laterally than on the corresponding CT, and in 13% of cases where the CT had shown extension through the posterior facet of the subtalar joint, the Broden view had falsely shown the fracture as projecting lateral to the joint.[33]

In the Sanders classification system of calcaneal fractures using CT, type I fractures are nondisplaced. Type II involve two separate articular fragments and are subdivided into A, B, and C types depending on the medial or lateral position of the fracture line

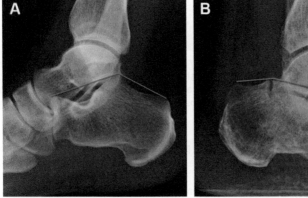

Fig. 17. (*A*) Normal Boehler angle on lateral radiograph. (*B*) Lateral radiograph in a patient with posttraumatic deformity with loss of Boehler angle.

through the posterior facet of the subtalar joint. Type III fractures have three separate articular fragments and are subdivided into AB, BC, and AC depending on the position of the fracture lines (**Fig. 18**). Type IV fractures have four or more separate articular surface fragments and thus are highly comminuted.[32] CT can also better identify the degree of displacement of the lateral calcaneal wall, and the presence of peroneal tendon entrapment within fracture fragments.

Fractures of the talus can also be commonly associated with subtalar joint dislocations. Isolated fractures of the talar neck can be classified with the Hawkins-Canale system for prognostic and treatment decisions depending on the association of subtalar and tibtiotalar dislocations.[34] Talar body fractures are usually comminuted and, in a recent retrospective series of 132 fractures using CT for primary diagnosis, talar body fractures were more commonly identified than talar neck fractures and were associated with subtalar joint subluxation or dislocation in 47% of cases (**Fig. 19**).[35]

The subtalar joint can be involved with arthritis, most commonly degenerative, but also inflammatory, infectious, and crystal deposition etiologies can occur. Radiographic detection of involvement of the subtalar joint in a cohort of patients with chronic rheumatoid arthritis with foot pain has been identified in 32% of these patients (**Fig. 20**).[36] MRI and ultrasound can increase detection of synovial inflammation in the hindfoot when compared with clinical examination.[37] Pigmented villonodular synovitis can involve the feet in 10% of cases, and in one of the larger patient series, subtalar joint involvement was usually seen with hindfoot presentation (**Fig. 21**).[38,39] Septic arthritis of the subtalar joint is also uncommon. It is rarely isolated to the subtalar joint, and with osteomyelitis of the calcaneus or associated infection of the tibiotalar joint more commonly seen (**Fig. 22**).[40]

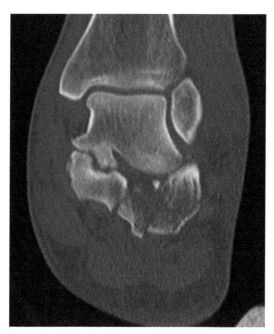

Fig. 18. Coronal reformatted CT image shows a comminuted Sanders type 3 AB calcaneal fracture with depression of the articular surface of the posterior subtalar joint. Note the abnormal broad undulating contour of the medial facet consistent with an incidental tarsal subtalar coalition.

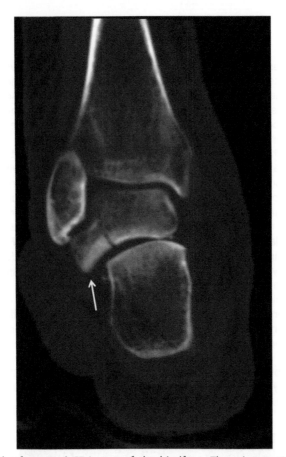

Fig. 19. Coronal reformatted CT image of the hindfoot. There is a posterior talar body fracture with lateral subluxation (*arrow*) of the posterior subtalar joint.

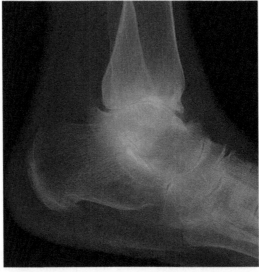

Fig. 20. Lateral radiograph of the hindfoot and ankle in a patient with long-standing rheumatoid arthritis. There is diffuse joint space loss on the tibiotalar and subtalar joint.

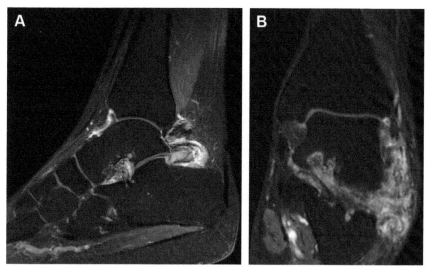

Fig. 21. MRI in a patient with pigmented villonodular synovitis of the subtalar joint. (*A*) Sagittal STIR shows distention of the posterior recess of the subtalar joint. Note decreased T2 signal within the synovial proliferative process consistent with hemosiderin deposition. (*B*) Coronal T2 fat-suppressed image shows the complex synovial process and erosive changes within the sinus tarsi.

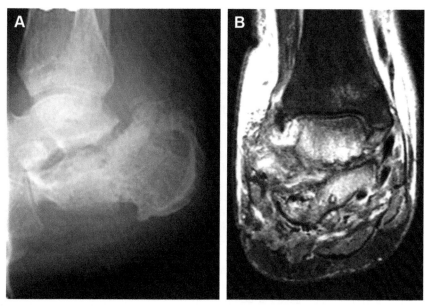

Fig. 22. Patient with septic subtalar joint. (*A*) Lateral radiograph shows marked erosive destruction of the subtalar joint with subchondral fragmentation. (*B*) Coronal STIR MRI of the same patient showing marked marrow edema of the talus and calcaneus and severe subcutaneous edema.

REFERENCES

1. Ayoob A, De Maeseneer M, Shahabpour M, et al. The talocalcaneal unit: pictorial review of anatomy and pathologic conditions on multi detector CT. JBR-BTR 2009;93(1):20–7.
2. Resnick D. Radiology of the talocalcaneal articulations: anatomic considerations and arthrography. Radiology 1974;111(3):581–6.
3. Bali N, Theivendran K, Prem H. Computed tomography review of tarsal canal anatomy with reference to the fitting of sinus tarsi implants in the tarsal canal. J Foot Ankle Surg 2013;52(6):714–6.
4. Klein MA, Spreitzer AM. MR imaging of the tarsal sinus and canal: normal anatomy, pathologic findings, and features of the sinus tarsi syndrome. Radiology 1993;186(1):233–40.
5. Beckly DE, Anderson PW, Pedegana LR. The radiology of the subtalar joint with special reference to talo-calcaneal coalition. Clin Radiol 1975;26:333–41.
6. Harris RI. Rigid valgus foot due to talocalcaneal bridge. J Bone Joint Surg Am 1955;37:169–82.
7. Drayer-Verhagen F. Arthritis of the subtalar joint associated with sustencalum tali facet configuration. J Anat 1993;183:631–4.
8. Lee MS, Harcke HT, Kumar SJ, et al. Subtalar joint coalition in children: new observations. Radiology 1989;172:635–9.
9. Liu PT, Roberts CC, Chivers FS, et al. "Absent middle facet": a sign on unenhanced radiography of subtalar joint coalition. AJR Am J Roentgenol 2003;181: 1565–72.
10. Isherwood I. A radiological approach to the subtalar joint. J Bone Joint Surg Br 1961;43(3):566–74.
11. Hirschmann A, Pfirrmann CW, Klammer G, et al. Upright cone CT of the hindfoot: comparison of the non-weight-bearing with the upright weight-bearing position. Eur Radiol 2014;24(3):553–8.
12. Sijbrandij ES, van Gils AP, de Lange EE, et al. Bone marrow ill-defined hyperintensities with tarsal coalition: MR imaging findings. Eur J Radiol 2002;43:61–5.
13. Jotoku T, Kinoshita M, Okuda R, et al. Anatomy of ligamentous structures in the tarsal sinus and canal. Foot Ankle Int 2006;27:533–8.
14. Linklater J, Hayter CL, Vu D, et al. Anatomy of the subtalar joint and imaging of talo-calcaneal coalition. Skeletal Radiol 2009;38:437–49.
15. Olson RW. Arthrography of the ankle: its use in the evaluation of ankle sprains. Radiology 1969;92:1439–46.
16. Goossens M, De Stoop N, Claessens H, et al. Posterior subtalar joint arthrography a useful tool in the diagnosis of hindfoot disorders. Clin Orthop Relat Res 1989;(249):248–55.
17. Sugimoto K, Samoto N, Takaoka T, et al. Subtalar arthrography in acute injuries of the calcane-ofibular ligament. J Bone Joint Surg Br 1998;80:785–90.
18. Ruhoy MK, Newberg AH, Yodlowski ML, et al. Subtalar joint arthrography. Semin Musculoskelet Radiol 1998;2(4):433–7.
19. Remedios D, Martin K, Kaplan G, et al. Juvenile chronic arthritis: diagnosis and management of tibiotalar and subtalar disease. Br J Rheumatol 1997;36:1214–7.
20. Smith J, Finnoff JT, Henning PT, et al. Accuracy of sonographically guided posterior subtalar joint injections comparison of 3 techniques. J Ultrasound Med 2009;28(11):1549–57.
21. Mosier KM. Tarsal coalitions and peroneal spastic flat foot—a review. J Bone Jt Surg Am 1984;66A:976–84.

22. Bohne WH. Tarsal coalition. Curr Opin Pediatr 2001;13:29–35.
23. Moe DC, Choi JJ, Davis KW. Posterior subtalar facet coalition with calcaneal stress fracture. AJR Am J Roentgenol 2006;186:259–64.
24. Kumar SJ, Guille JT, Lee MS, et al. Osseous and non-osseous coalition of the middle facet of the talocalcaneal joint. J Bone Joint Surg Am 1992;74:529–35.
25. Wechsler RJ, Karasick D, Schweitzer ME. Computed tomography of talocalaneal coalition: imaging techniques. Skeletal Radiol 1992;21:353–8.
26. Crim JR, Kjeldsberg KM. Radiographic diagnosis of tarsal coalition. AJR Am J Roentgenol 2004;182:323–8.
27. Resnick D. Talar ridges, osteophytes, and beaks: a radiologic commentary. Radiology 1984;151:329–32.
28. Lateur LM, Van Hoe LR, Van Ghillewe KV, et al. Subtalar coalition: diagnosis with the C sign on lateral radiographs of the ankle. Radiology 1994;193:847–51.
29. Nalaboff KM, Schweitzer ME. MRI of tarsal coalition: frequency, distribution, and innovative signs. Bull NYU Hosp Jt Dis 2008;66:14–21.
30. Bianchi S, Hoffman D. Ultrasound of talocalcaneal coalition: retrospective study of 11 patients. Skeletal Radiol 2013;42:1209–14.
31. Daftary A, Haims AH, Baumgaertner M. Fractures of the calcaneus: a review with emphasis on CT. Radiographics 2005;25:1215–26.
32. Sanders R. Displaced intra-articular fractures of the calcaneus. J Bone Joint Surg Am 2000;82(2):225–50.
33. Kwon DG, Chung CY, Lee KM, et al. Revisit of Broden's view for intraarticular calcaneal fracture. Clin Orthop Surg 2012;4(3):221–6.
34. Canale ST, Kelly FB Jr. Fractures of the neck of the talus. J Bone Joint Surg Am 1978;60:143–56.
35. Dale JD, Ha AS, Chew FS. Update on talar fracture patterns: a large level I trauma center study. Am J Roentgenol 2013;201(5):1087–92.
36. Vidigal E, Jacoby RK, Dixon AS, et al. The foot in chronic rheumatoid arthritis. Ann Rheum Dis 1975;34(4):292–7.
37. Wakefield RJ, Freeston JE, O'Connor P, et al. The optimal assessment of the rheumatoid arthritis hindfoot: a comparative study of clinical examination, ultrasound and high field MRI. Ann Rheum Dis 2008;67(8):1678–82.
38. Ghert MA, Scully SP, Harrelson JM. Pigmented villonodular synovitis of the foot and ankle: a review of six cases. Foot Ankle Int 1999;20:326–30.
39. Brien EW, Sacoman DM, Mirra JM. Pigmented villonodular synovitis of the foot and ankle. Foot Ankle Int 2004;25(12):908–13.
40. Wynes J, Harris W IV, Hadfield RA, et al. Subtalar joint septic arthritis in a patient with hypogammaglobulinemia. J Foot Ankle Surg 2013;52(2):242–8.

Subtalar Instability

Michael Aynardi, MD[a], David I. Pedowitz, MD[a],
Steven M. Raikin, MD[b],*

KEYWORDS

- Subtalar joint • Subtalar instability • Ankle instability • Subtalar dislocation

KEY POINTS

- Subtalar instability is difficult to diagnose and is often overlooked as a component of traditional ankle instability.
- Clinicians should have a high index of suspicion of this diagnosis in patients who have been diagnosed with chronic lateral ankle instability but have failed standard management and have continued pain in the sinus tarsi.
- Operative management includes ligamentous reconstruction of key lateral stabilizers of the subtalar joint.

INTRODUCTION

Although often overlooked and grouped into the larger clinical entity of ankle instability, an unstable subtalar joint is a relatively common clinical entity occurring in approximately one-quarter of all cases of chronic lateral ankle instability.[1] When considering that chronic ankle instability occurs in nearly 20% of all patients sustaining inversion injuries to the foot and ankle,[2] one may appreciate the importance of identifying and addressing this condition.

ANATOMY AND BIOMECHANICAL ANALYSIS

The subtalar joint describes the articulation between the calcaneus and talus. The bony anatomy of the joint is composed of 3 articulating facets: posterior, middle, and anterior. In concert, these glide in 3 different planes of motion to produce inversion/eversion, abduction/adduction, and flexion/extension.[3] The motion of the subtalar joint occurs about a center of rotation that is positioned $42 \pm 9°$ of inclination in the sagittal

The authors have nothing to disclose.
[a] Department of Orthopaedic Surgery, Rothman Institute of Orthopaedics, Thomas Jefferson University Hospital, Philadelphia, PA 19107, USA; [b] Foot and Ankle Service, Rothman Institute of Orthopaedics, Thomas Jefferson University Hospital, 925 Chestnut Street, 5th Floor, Philadelphia, PA 19107, USA
* Corresponding author.
E-mail address: steven.raikin@rothmaninstitute.com

plane and $23 \pm 11°$ of medial deviation in the horizontal plane relative to the axis of the foot passing through the second web space of the foot.[4] In concert, these articulations are responsible for stability and accommodation when walking on uneven ground.

Reported range of motion (ROM) of the subtalar joint varies widely in the literature and is largely thought of as motion specifically at the posterior facet. Sarrafian[5] initially reported a ROM of 25° of inversion/supination and 10° of eversion/pronation. Meanwhile, others have demonstrated positioning of the ankle joint impacts the measured ROM of the joint.[6] Last, clinical subtalar motion, as measured by goniometer, may vary from radiographic measurements. Pearce and Buckley[7] demonstrated a large difference in clinical measurement, mean 46° (range, 39–54) as compared with measurements using computed tomography, mean 11° (range, 5–16), which they concluded was the result of soft tissue and talocrural motion.

The lateral ligamentous structures of the subtalar joint are organized in layers. The superficial layer includes the calcaneofibular ligament (CFL), the lateral talocalcaneal ligament, and the lateral root of the inferior retinaculum. The middle layer is composed of the cervical ligament and the intermediate root of the retinaculum, and the deep layer is formed by the interosseous talocalcaneal ligament (ITCL) and medial root of retinaculum.[8]

Etiologies for subtalar instability include the cervical ligament, the CFL, and the ITCL. Historically, the CFL was recognized as the primary ligamentous stabilizer to the subtalar joint.[9] However, a large body of evidence now supports the ITCL as the primary stabilizer to the subtalar joint.[10–12] Recently, Choisne and colleagues[10] reported the greatest increase in subtalar joint instability with sectioning of the ITCL with the foot dorsiflexed, supinated, and inverted. These findings are consistent with the hypothesis that rupture of the ITCL and cervical ligament occur during subtalar dislocation, as described previously by several investigators.[13–16] Moreover, the ITCL appears to play a role in ankle stability in addition to the subtalar joint. Tochigi and colleagues[17] demonstrated that combined sectioning of the ITCL and anterior talofibular ligament (ATFL) resulted in an anterolateral rotatory displacement of the talus, whereas isolated sectioning of the ATFL did not. The investigators conducted a follow-up study investigating ITCL injuries in acute ankle sprains and found a correlation between persistent symptoms of lateral ankle pain, instability, and limitation of motion with ITCL injuries on MRI.[18] These studies help underscore the importance of the ITCL in hind foot stability.

CLINICAL PRESENTATION

Patients with subtalar instability generally provide a history of an acute inversion injury to the ankle in the past. Typically, they report multiple recurrent events. Initially diagnosed and treated for an ankle sprain, these patients are managed conservatively and often return with vague complaints of lateral pain about the ankle and hind foot that is worse with activity, especially athletics or activity on uneven ground. The pain often may be nonspecific and diffuse. Patients report symptoms of instability, including a feeling of the ankle "giving way" or "rolling over." Occasionally, patients may state they must look at the ground because they are unsure of their footing. In addition, patients may report lateral ankle swelling and stiffness.[19,20] Unfortunately, the presentation of this entity is nearly impossible to differentiate from lateral ankle instability.

PHYSICAL EXAMINATION

The signs of subtalar instability on physical examination mirror lateral ankle instability. Depending on the chronicity of the injury, patients may have lateral swelling, ecchymosis, and tenderness to palpation, often in the sinus tarsi. Unlike patients with isolated ankle instability, as swelling subsides, patients with subtalar instability will have persistent sinus tarsi pain. They often demonstrate increased inversion on hind foot stress examination as well as a positive anterior drawer when the CFL is disrupted.[21,22] A specific test for subtalar instability testing for chronic anterolateral rotatory instability of the subtalar joint was described by Thermann and colleagues.[21] In this test, the examiner holds the heel and forefoot rigid with the foot in 10° of dorsiflexion. First, an inversion and internal rotation stress is applied followed by an adduction stress to the forefoot (**Fig. 1**). A positive examination results in a medial shift of the calcaneus under the talus, as well as an opening of the talocalcaneal angle. Furthermore, the investigators validated this examination maneuver radiographically in a study using Broden views. The investigators report a positive examination is defined by greater than 5 mm of medial calcaneal displacement or greater than 5° of talocalcaneal tilt.

IMAGING

Initial evaluation should include standing radiographs of the ankle or hind foot. Many investigators once advocated for inversion stress examination using a Broden view on either radiographs or tomography to diagnose subtalar instability. First described by Rubin and Witten[13] and supported by Brantigan and colleagues,[1] these studies show an increase in subtalar inversion of almost 20° between symptomatic individuals and controls. Several investigators developed various radiographic criteria for diagnosing subtalar instability. Heilman and colleagues[15] used separation of the posterior facet of the calcaneus and talus over 7 mm after sectioning of the CFL and ITCL in cadavers to define subtalar instability radiographically. However, both Louwerens and colleagues[23] and Harper[24] were unable to support the use of these stress examinations, as they failed to establish a correlation between radiographic findings and clinical symptoms.

Using different stress techniques, Kato[25] performed anterior stress radiographs that measured displacement of the calcaneus relative to the talus. In this series, the

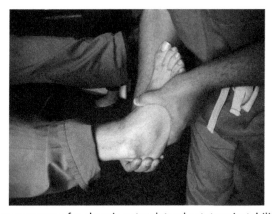

Fig. 1. Examination maneuver for chronic anterolateral rotatory instability of the subtalar joint. In this test, the examiner holds the heel and forefoot rigid with the foot in 10° of dorsiflexion. First, an inversion and internal rotation stress is applied followed by an adduction stress to the forefoot. A positive examination results in a medial shift of the calcaneus under the talus.

investigators reported an increase in anterior translation of the calcaneus averaging 5 mm in all 50 patients who were diagnosed clinically with subtalar instability (**Fig. 2**).

In addition to radiographs, other imaging modalities have been used to aid in the diagnosis of subtalar instability. Through the use of dynamic ultrasound, Waldecker and Blatter[26] measured the fibula-trochlear angle in neutral position and under inversion stress to demonstrate an unstable subtalar joint. The investigators reported sonographic ratios of greater than 1.6 between positions as diagnostic for subtalar instability. Other investigators have explored the use of subtalar arthrography to evaluate the subtalar joint. Both Meyer and colleagues[14] and Sugimoto and colleagues[27] have reported the effectiveness at diagnosing ruptures to ligamentous structures of the subtalar joint. Additionally, MRI has been used to evaluate the ligamentous structures of the subtalar joint. Tochigi and colleagues[18] were able to demonstrate a relationship between injury to the ITCL and clinical symptoms of instability and pain in patients with subtalar instability. Recently, Seebauer and colleagues[28] described the use of MRI stress examination to aid in the diagnosis of subtalar and ankle instability. In their series, they compared symptomatic individuals with controls and were able to show accurate assessment of multiple parameters of subtalar and ankle instability with objective imaging. Additionally, they cite the advantage of stress examination with MRI as a way for a simultaneous direct comparison of laxity for both the subtalar and ankle joints.

ARTHROSCOPY

Ankle arthroscopy can also be helpful as an aid to diagnosing subtalar instability. In a retrospective review of patients undergoing subtalar joint arthroscopy, Frey and

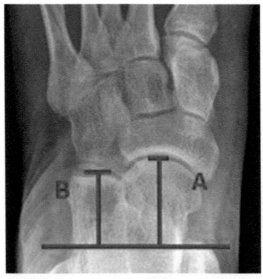

Fig. 2. An anteroposterior radiograph centered over the talonavicular joint to assess for subtalar instability. First, the talomalleolar distance, A, and the calcano malleolar distance are measured, B. Traction in line with the foot is applied under stress radiograph and the measurements are repeated. A difference in anterior translation greater than 5 mm, subtalar displacement = $(B_{Stress} - B_{Rest}) - (A_{Stress} - A_{Rest})$, is considered significant for subtalar instability. (*Adapted from* Kato T. The diagnosis and treatment of instability of the subtalar joint. J Bone Joint Surg Br 1995;77:401.)

colleagues[29] were able to accurately identify an ITCL tear as the cause for instability in 36 of 45 patients. Hence, arthroscopy may be helpful in cases in which history, examination, and imaging are equivocal.

TREATMENT

Once the diagnosis of subtalar instability has been established, nonoperative management should be initiated. Similar to ankle instability, physical therapy, bracing, and proper shoe wear are all first-line treatments for subtalar instability. The goals of physical therapy are to strengthen the soft tissue stabilizers surrounding the ankle and subtalar joint as well as improve flexibility of the Achilles to allow for better hind foot positioning.[30] In cases of deformity, orthotics is often helpful at preventing malpositioning of the subtalar joint.[31] Recently, Choisne and colleagues[32] evaluated the effects of a semirigid ankle brace on simulated subtalar motion. Kinematics from 9 cadaveric feet was collected in various foot positions both with and without a brace. The investigators sequentially sectioned the CFL and the intrinsic ligaments. They found that isolated CFL sectioning only increased ankle joint inversion, whereas sectioning both the CFL and intrinsic ligaments affected subtalar joint stability. They also demonstrated that simulations in the semirigid brace limited inversion at both the subtalar and ankle joints. They concluded that bracing may be beneficial in patients with subtalar instability.

Operative management is indicated in symptomatic individuals who fail conservative treatment. Surgical reconstruction of the subtalar joint for instability is aimed at restoring the key stabilizers of the joint: the ITCL, CFL, and cervical ligament. Several surgical techniques have been described for instability of the subtalar joint.[33–40] One of the earliest procedures was by Elmslie[33] and involved a reconstruction of the CFL and ATFL with a fascia lata graft. Chrisman and Snook[36] used a similar technique but used one-half of peroneus brevis. Using their technique they reported a small series of 7 patients with instability, 3 of the 7 had documented subtalar instability, which were all able to return to previous levels of activity. Although these reconstructions function as a checkrein to inversion of the subtalar joint, they are not anatomic in their reconstruction of the ligaments and may lead to stiffness and possibly arthritis in the long term.[34,37] In addition, Larsen[37] used the entire peroneus brevis tendon through a V-shaped tunnel in the fibula to reconstruct the lateral ligaments. In that series, 71 of 79 ankles had resolution of radiographic ankle instability postoperative. Although not statistically significant, Larsen[37] noted a reduction in subtalar supination as well. Last, Larsen[37] noted return to sporting activities in all patients.

Other investigators have described a triligamentous reconstruction of the lateral ligamentous structures using a variety of graft materials through bone tunnels. Schon and colleagues[34] described a weave of the plantaris or entire peroneus brevis through a lateral tunnel in the calcaneus, into the tarsal canal, through a tunnel in the talar neck, through the fibula, then into a posterior calcaneal tunnel. Kato[25] described reconstruction of the ITCL anatomically by using a partial Achilles tendon graft, reporting good results in 12 patients undergoing triligamentous reconstruction with this technique. Recently Jung and Kim[41] demonstrated a novel reconstruction using a semitendinosus allograft using a 2-limbed weave. The anterior portion recreates the ITCL and cervical ligaments and the posterior limb reconstructing the CFL. Advantages of this technique include anatomic reconstruction without sacrificing a dynamic lateral stabilizer, the peroneus brevis, and it is technically less demanding than other reconstructions (**Fig. 3**). Other investigators have described ligamentous reconstruction with arthroscopic assistance for visualization of tunnel placement by using a gracilis tendon from the ipsilateral knee.

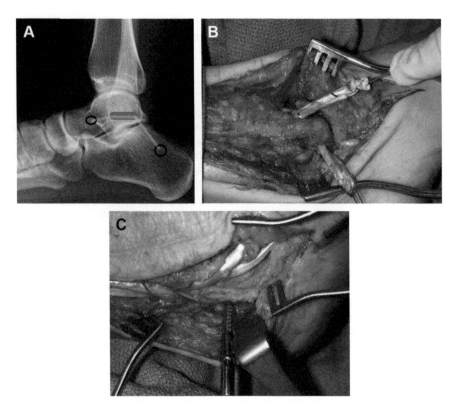

Fig. 3. (*A*) Preoperative planning radiographs demonstrating tunnel placement and position for graft fixation at the talar footprint, the fibular bone tunnel, and calcaneal bone tunnel. (*B*) Intraoperative photograph after passage of semitendinosus allograft. (*C*) Interference screw fixation of the calcaneal limb of the graft under tension.

ACUTE SUBTALAR DISLOCATION

Although rare, acute subtalar dislocation can result in subtalar instability. These injuries are common in men in their third decade of life and occur via a supinated hindfoot sustaining an inversion force usually resulting in a medial dislocation (**Fig. 4**).[42] It has been theorized by Keefe and Haddad[19] that the injury to the lateral structures of the ankle occurs in the following order: CFL, lateral talocalcaneal ligament, the cervical ligament, and last the ITCL. Treatment of these dislocations through immediate closed reduction in the emergency room with anesthesia is often successful. Reduction is achieved by flexing the knee to relax the gastrocnemius while the surgeon first accentuates the deformity, then applies longitudinal traction, and finally reverses the deformity. If closed attempts are unsuccessful, open reduction is indicated. Typically, a mechanical block to reduction is present, which may be caused by interposition of the posterior tibial tendon for a lateral dislocation or interposition of the extensor digitorum brevis muscle for medial dislocations.[42] After reduction, patients are often treated with some form of immobilization and are made full weight bearing in a walker boot or walking cast for 4 to 6 weeks. Physical therapy is then initiated for improvement of strength, ROM, and proprioception. Although chronic instability has been reported following subtalar dislocations, the progression of posttraumatic arthritis after

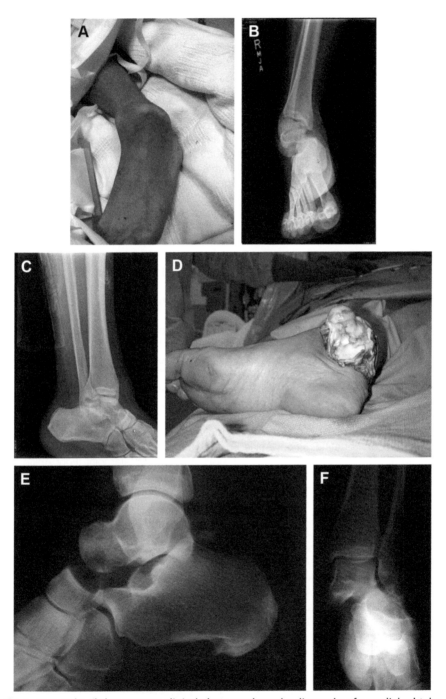

Fig. 4. Images (*A–C*) demonstrate clinical photographs and radiographs of a medial subtalar dislocation. Images (*D–F*) show an open lateral subtalar dislocation that required open reduction and irrigation and debridement in the operating room.

these injuries is common and often results in worse clinical outcome when compared with the noninjured limb.[43] Additionally, dislocations that require open reduction result in poor clinical outcomes.[44]

SUMMARY

Although often difficult to diagnose and is overlooked as a component of traditional ankle instability, subtalar instability is a common clinical entity. In particular, clinicians should have a high index of suspicion of this diagnosis in patients who have been diagnosed with chronic lateral ankle instability but have failed standard management and have continued pain in the sinus tarsi. As with ankle instability, nonoperative management is the initial mainstay of treatment. Operative management includes ligamentous reconstruction of key lateral stabilizers of the subtalar joint. Future research on this subject should be focused at improving diagnosis and recognition of this entity.

REFERENCES

1. Brantigan JW, Pedegana LR, Lippert FG. Instability of the subtalar joint. Diagnosis by stress tomography in three cases. J Bone Joint Surg Am 1977;59:321–4.
2. Freeman MA. Instability of the foot after injuries to the lateral ligament of the ankle. J Bone Joint Surg Br 1965;47:669–77.
3. Perry J. Anatomy and biomechanics of the hindfoot. Clin Orthop 1983;177:9–15.
4. Inman VT. The joints of the ankle. Philadelphia: Williams & Wilkins; 1976.
5. Sarrafian SK. Biomechanics of the subtalar joint complex. Clin Orthop Relat Res 1993;(290):17–26.
6. Milgrom C, Giladi M, Simkin A, et al. The normal range of subtalar inversion and eversion in young males as measured by three different techniques. Foot Ankle Int 1985;6:143–5.
7. Pearce TJ, Buckley RE. Subtalar joint movement: clinical and computed tomography scan correlation. Foot Ankle Int 1999;20:428–32.
8. Harper MC. The lateral ligamentous support of the subtalar joint. Foot Ankle Int 1991;11:354–8.
9. Kjaersgaard-Andersen P, Wethelund JO, Nielsen S. Lateral talocalcaneal instability following section of the calcaneofibular ligament: a kinesiologic study. Foot Ankle Int 1987;7:355–61.
10. Choisne J, Ringleb S, Samaan MA, et al. Influence of kinematic analysis methods on detecting ankle and subtalar joint instability. J Biomech 2012;45:46–52.
11. Ringleb SI, Dhakal A, Anderson CD, et al. Effects of lateral ligament sectioning on the stability of the ankle and subtalar joint. J Orthop Res 2011;29:1459–64.
12. Tochigi Y, Amendola A, Rudert MJ, et al. The role of the interosseous talocalcaneal ligament in subtalar joint stability. Foot Ankle Int 2004;25:588–96.
13. Rubin G, Witten M. The subtalar joint and the symptom of turning over on the ankle: a new method of evaluation utilizing tomography. Am J Orthop 1962;4:16–9.
14. Meyer JM, Garcia J, Hoffmeyer P, et al. The subtalar sprain. A roentgenographic study. Clin Orthop Relat Res 1988;(226):169–73.
15. Heilman AE, Braly WG, Bishop JO, et al. An anatomic study of subtalar instability. Foot Ankle Int 1990;10:224–8.
16. Bonnel F, Toullec E, Mabit C, et al. Chronic ankle instability: biomechanics and pathomechanics of ligaments injury and associated lesions. Orthop Traumatol Surg Res 2010;96:424–32.

17. Tochigi Y, Takahashi K, Yamagata M, et al. Influence of the interosseous talocal-caneal ligament injury on stability of the ankle subtalar joint complex—a cadaveric experimental study. Foot Ankle Int 2000;21:486–91.
18. Tochigi Y, Yoshinaga K, Wada Y, et al. Acute inversion injury of the ankle: magnetic resonance imaging and clinical outcomes. Foot Ankle Int 1998;19:730–4.
19. Keefe DT, Haddad SL. Subtalar instability. Etiology, diagnosis, and management. Foot Ankle Clin 2002;7:577–609.
20. Karlsson J, Eriksson B, Renstrom P. Subtalar ankle instability. Sports Med 1997; 24:337–46.
21. Thermann H, Zwipp H, Tscherne H. Treatment algorithm for chronic ankle and subtalar instability. Foot Ankle Int 1997;18:163–9.
22. Mann RA. Athletic injuries to the soft tissues of the foot and ankle. In: Mann RA, Coughlin MJ, editors. Surgery of the foot and ankle. 7th edition. St Louis (MO): Mosby; 1999. p. 1153–65.
23. Louwerens JW, Ginai AZ, van Linge B, et al. Stress radiography of the talocrural and subtalar joints. Foot Ankle Int 1995;16:148–55.
24. Harper MC. Stress radiographs in the diagnosis of lateral instability of the ankle and hindfoot. Foot Ankle Int 1993;13:435–8.
25. Kato T. The diagnosis and treatment of instability of the subtalar joint. J Bone Joint Surg Br 1995;77:400–6.
26. Waldecker U, Blatter G. Sonographic measurement of instability of the subtalar joint. Foot Ankle Int 2001;22:42–6.
27. Sugimoto K, Samoto N, Takaoka T, et al. Subtalar arthrography in acute injuries of the calcaneofibular ligament. J Bone Joint Surg Br 1998;80:785–90.
28. Seebauer C, Bail H, Rump JC, et al. Ankle laxity: stress investigation under MRI control. AJR Am J Roentgenol 2013;201:496–504.
29. Frey C, Feder KS, DiGiovanni C. Arthroscopic evaluation of the subtalar joint: does sinus tarsi syndrome exist? Foot Ankle Int 1999;20:185–91.
30. Clanton TO. Instability of the subtalar joint. Orthop Clin North Am 1989;20: 583–92.
31. LoPiccolo M, Chilvers M, Graham B, et al. Effectiveness of the cavus foot orthosis. J Surg Orthop Adv 2010;19:166–9.
32. Choisne J, Hoch M, Bawab S, et al. The effects of a semi-rigid ankle brace on a simulated isolated subtalar joint instability. J Orthop Res 2013;31:1869–75.
33. Elmslie RC. Recurrent subluxation of the ankle joint. Ann Surg 1934;100:364–7.
34. Schon LC, Clanton TO, Baxter DE. Reconstruction for subtalar instability: a review. Foot Ankle 1991;11:319–25.
35. Karlsson J, Bergsten T, Lansinger O, et al. Reconstruction of the lateral ligaments of the ankle for chronic lateral instability. J Bone Joint Surg Am 1988;70(4):581–8.
36. Chrisman OD, Snook G. Reconstruction of lateral ligament tears of the ankle: an experimental study and clinical evaluation of seven patients treated by a new modification of the Elmslie procedure. J Bone Joint Surg Am 1969;51A:904–12.
37. Larsen E. Tendon transfer for lateral ankle and subtalar joint instability. Acta Orthop Scand 1988;59(2):168–72.
38. Lui TH. Arthroscopic-assisted lateral ligamentous reconstruction in combined ankle and subtalar instability. Arthroscopy 2007;23(5):554–5.
39. Pisani G. Chronic laxity of the subtalar joint. Orthopedics 1996;19(5):431–7.
40. Pagenstert GI, Hintermann B, Knupp M. Operative management of chronic ankle instability: plantaris graft. Foot Ankle Clin 2006;11(3):567–83.
41. Jung H, Kim T. Subtalar instability reconstruction with an allograft: technical note. Foot Ankle Int 2012;33:682–5.

42. Delee JC, Curtis R. Subtalar dislocation of the foot. J Bone Joint Surg Am 1982; 64:433–7.
43. Bibbo C, Anderson RB, Davis WH. Injury characteristics and the clinical outcome of subtalar dislocations: a clinical and radiographic analysis of 25 cases. Foot Ankle Int 2003;24:158–63.
44. Woodruff MJ, Brown JN, Mountney J. A mechanism for entrapment of the tibialis posterior tendon in lateral subtalar dislocation. Injury 1996;27:193–4.

Subtalar Dislocations

Stefan Rammelt, MD, PhD*, Jens Goronzy, MD

KEYWORDS

- Subtalar joint • Dislocation • Talar process fracture • Avascular necrosis
- Open dislocation

KEY POINTS

- Treatment of subtalar dislocations consists of early reduction under adequate sedation or open reduction if necessary.
- Purely ligamentous subtalar dislocations have an excellent prognosis with early reduction.
- Complications such as avascular necrosis and posttraumatic arthritis are seen predominately after open dislocations, total talar dislocations, and associated fractures.

Subtalar dislocation (syn.: luxatio pedis sub talo) is defined as a simultaneous dislocation of the subtalar (talocalcaneal) and talonavicular joints. The first case report was probably provided by DuFaurest in 1811.[1] Broca, in 1853, termed them "luxations sous-astragaliennes" and he discriminated between medial, lateral, and posterior dislocations, in descending order of frequency.[2] Malgaigne[3] and Henke[4] later added an anterior type. With this modification, Broca's classification of subtalar dislocations is still in use today. Leitner, in an analysis of 4521 dislocations at Böhler's clinic in 1952, found 42 cases of subtalar dislocations (36 medial, 6 lateral) and brought attention to the fact that interposed ligaments and tendons may warrant open reduction.[5]

Subtalar dislocations have to be distinguished from tibiotalar (ankle) dislocations (luxatio pedis cum talo), midtarsal (Chopart) dislocations that involve the talonavicular and calcaneocuboid joint, and total talar dislocations (luxatio tali totalis) from the ankle and subtalar joints.[6] Subtalar dislocations represent between 1% and 2% of all dislocations and 15% of all peritalar injuries.[7] They occur more frequently in men than in women and predominately affect people in their mid-30s.[8,9] Although pure ligamentous dislocations have an excellent prognosis after proper reduction, care has to be taken not to overlook the frequent associated bony injuries like fractures of the lateral talar process and the sustentaculum tali that may rapidly lead to the development of painful posttraumatic arthritis of the subtalar joint.[10–12]

The authors have nothing to disclose.
Foot & Ankle Section, University Center for Orthopaedics and Traumatology, TU Dresden, University Hospital Carl Gustav Carus, Dresden, Germany
* Corresponding author. Universitäts Centrum für Orthopädie und Unfallchirurgie, Universitätsklinikum "Carl Gustav Carus" der TU Dresden, Fetscherstrasse 74, Dresden 01307, Germany.
E-mail address: stefan.rammelt@uniklinikum-dresden.de

RELEVANT ANATOMY

The subtalar joint is divided by the strong talocalcaneal ligaments in the sinus tarsi and the tarsal canal into an anterior and posterior portion. The latter is formed by the posterior joint facets of the talus and calcaneus and is saddle shaped. The anterior portion forms a functional unit with the talonavicular joint (talcalcaneonavicular joint). It is a ball-and-socket joint that has also been called "coxa pedis" because of the developmental and functional similarities with the hip.

The subtalar joint is stabilized by its inherent bony structure and reinforced by numerous ligaments at the sinus tarsi, the tarsal canal, the posterior subtalar joint, and the talonavicular joint. An important stabilizer for the subtalar joint is the ligament complex in the sinus and canalis tarsi, the components of which display a substantial variability and are termed inconsistently in the literature. Schmidt, who gave one of the most detailed descriptions of the complex anatomy of the ligaments in the sinus tarsi and tarsal canal in 1978, discriminates 5 separate ligaments that form the complex of the interosseous ligament (IOL): the lateral, intermediate and medial roots of the inferior extensor retinacle (IER), the oblique talocalcaneal ligament (also referred to as cervical ligament because it connects the talar neck with the calcaneal neck), and the talocalcaneal interosseous ligament (TCIL) which he also termed the ligament of the tarsal canal.[13] He stated that 4 of the 5 parts limit excessive supination and inversion because they lie laterally to the pivot of the subtalar joint, whereas only the medial root of the IER limits pronation and eversion. Several authors have described a V-shaped appearance of the TCIL, and 2 recent studies on 40[14] and 32 cadaver feet[15] noted that the fibers of the TCIL blend with those of the medial root of the IER, forming a V-shaped ligament. Li and colleagues[15] in addition identified a smaller, separate tarsal canal ligament anterior to this complex and behind the medial subtalar joint facets in 20 of 32 specimens; Jotoku and colleagues[14] termed it the "anterior capsular ligament."

The important calcaneofibular ligament, running form the tip of the fibula to the posterior part of the calcaneal tuberosity, provides lateral stability to both the ankle and subtalar joints.[16] Smaller, inconstant ligaments (lateral and posterior talocalcaneal ligaments) are merely capsular reinforcements. Recently, Li and colleagues[15] identified a posterior capsular ligament in 25 of 32 specimens directly in front of the posterior facet of the subtalar joint. On the medial side, the ligamentous support for the subtalar joint is provided by the tibiocalcaneal ligament as a part of the deltoid ligament complex.[6,17]

The bifurcate ligament stabilizes both the anterior portion of the subtalar joint (the talocalcaneonavicular joint) and the midtarsal (Chopart's) joint. The common origin of both the calcaneonavicular and calcaneocuboidal parts of the bifurcate ligament lies on the dorsal aspect of the anterior process of the calcaneus. According to Schmidt and Grünwald[18] the calcaneonavicular part is stronger with an average diameter of 3 mm and longer with an average length of 15 mm than the calcaneocuboidal part (2 and 9 mm, respectively). The anterior subtalar (talocalcaneonavicular) joint is further stabilized by the dorsal talonavicular ligaments (mainly capsule reinforcements), the strong plantar calcaneonavicular ("Spring") ligament and medial calcaneonavicular (Volkmann's "neglected") ligament.[19]

MECHANISM OF INJURY

Because of the strong ligamentous support, subtalar dislocations are caused by high-energy injuries like motor vehicle accidents and falls from a height in 50% to 80% of cases.[20–22] However, a substantial number of subtalar dislocations result from rather trivial injuries or during sports ("basketball foot").[23] In a recent literature review of 359 subtalar dislocations, 44% were caused by a traffic accident, 33% by a fall, and 14% by sports injuries.[9]

Medial subtalar dislocations make up about 75% of all reported cases.[5,7,9] They are produced by forced inversion of the plantarflexed foot with the sustentaculum tali serving as a lever for the talar neck. The lateral talonavicular ligaments are the first to rupture, followed by the subtalar ligaments that rupture from medial to lateral.[6] In contrast, lateral subtalar dislocations make up 17% to 26% of the reported cases in larger series and are produced by forced eversion with the foot in dorsiflexion.[5,7,9] The anterior process of the calcaneus acts as a fulcrum for the lateral edge of the talar head.[24] Beside the talonavicular and interosseous ligaments, the deltoid ligament is frequently ruptured in these conditions. If the forces leading to medial or lateral subtalar dislocations continue, tibiotalar subluxation or complete talar dislocation may occur.[5] The calcaneocuboid ligaments usually remain intact, but in rare cases the calcaneocuboid joint may be dislocated too, resulting in a "peritalar dislocation."[25] Posterior and anterior dislocations are rare, making up 2% and 1% of all subtalar dislocations, respectively.[7,9] Posterior subtalar dislocations are caused by heavy plantarflexion of the foot, and anterior subtalar dislocations are most likely produced by anterior traction of the foot with the lower leg being fixed.[26–29]

Leitner[5] regarded subtalar dislocations as a first stage to total talar dislocations. The latter would result from continuing force including inversion stress on the ankle joint in medial or lateral dislocations. Repetitive subluxation may lead to recurrent subtalar sprains and chronic instability with constant stress, like in ballet dancers. Menetrey and Fritschy[30] reported on 25 subluxations of the talonavicular and subtalar joints in members of 1 ballet company within 1 year.

DIAGNOSIS

Dislocation of the foot beneath the talus in medial and lateral subtalar dislocation is usually obvious (**Fig. 1**A). Medial dislocations result in a medially displaced heel, inversion, and plantarflexion of the foot. The skin is tented over the prominent talar head and lateral malleolus. Lateral dislocations are typically high-energy injuries and are more frequently associated with open injuries. The heel is displaced laterally and the foot is in inversion and abduction. The talar head is visible and palpable medially (see **Fig. 1**B). The deformity is less marked in posterior or anterior dislocations

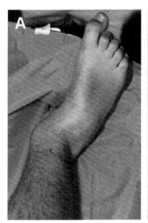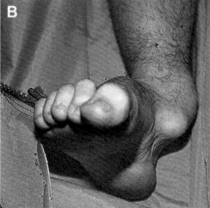

Fig. 1. (*A, B*) Clinical appearance of a lateral subtalar dislocation with the foot lateral to the lower leg and a medially prominent talar head.

because there is less axial malalignment, but the vulnerable skin over the foot may be tented.[21] The foot and ankle are checked for open injuries, critical soft tissue conditions, and neurovascular deficits. The diagnosis is confirmed with anteroposterior and lateral radiographs. With the dislocated foot, the projections will not be correct, but the direction of dislocation and associated fractures can be estimated (**Fig. 2**). Successful reduction is documented with fluoroscopy or standard radiographs (**Fig. 3**). Because subtalar dislocations are associated with talar process fractures and other peritalar injuries in more than 60% of cases, CT is advised after closed or open reduction (**Fig. 4**) to not miss relevant injuries on plain radiographs.[10]

TREATMENT

Early reduction of subtalar dislocations is warranted to avoid further damage to the soft tissues and neurovascular compromise. If performed promptly, the majority of subtalar dislocations can be reduced in a closed manner under sedation; delayed reduction may require general anesthesia and proper relaxation. The patient's knee is bent 90° to minimize the pull of the gastrocnemius–soleus complex on the heel. As in most dislocations, reduction starts with traction and accentuation followed by reversal of the deformity. Direct pressure on the palpable, prominent talar head facilitates reduction.

For medial subtalar dislocations, the foot is plantarflexed, inverted, and pulled distally to unlock the talar head from the navicular. One hand holds the tibia from the front and the other hand holds the heel from the back. The foot is then dorsiflexed and everted with direct pressure from lateral on the prominent talar head. Successful reduction is accompanied by an audible click. In approximately 10% of medial subtalar dislocations, closed reduction is impossible. The talar head may be incarcerated into the superior extensor retinacle (ligamentum cruciatum) or the bellies of the extensor digitorum brevis muscle like in a buttonhole. Other, rare obstacles to closed reduction include the talonavicular joint capsule, the deep posterior neurovascular bundle, or the peroneal tendons.[8,24,31] Locked dislocations of the navicular within the talar neck owing to direct impaction have also been described.[10] In these cases, open reduction via an anterolateral or oblique (Ollier's) lateral approach directly over the palpable talar head is indicated. The talar head is freed gently with direct manipulation or using a smooth elevator and finally the subtalar joint can be reduced manually. Incarcerated small avulsed bony fragments are removed.

For closed reduction of lateral subtalar dislocations, both the hip and knee are flexed about 90°. The foot is brought in dorsiflexion and eversion and pulled distally. Reduction is then completed with plantarflexion and inversion of the foot beneath the talus. Medial pressure is applied to the talar head. In up to 40% of reported cases the tibialis posterior or—more rarely—the flexor digitorum longus tendon is slung around the talar head and prevents closed reduction. In these instances, open reduction via a direct incision over the prominent talar head becomes necessary. The tibialis posterior tendon, which is slung around the talar head laterally, is pushed back medially with a smooth elevator. Reduction of the subtalar joint is then achieved by pulling the foot anteriorly and medially. After reduction, the lateral talar process should be inspected for an associated fracture or interposed bony or cartilaginous avulsions. Larger fragments of the lateral process are reduced anatomically and fixed with small (2.0–2.7 mm) screws. Smaller or multiple fragments are resected. Displaced fractures of the posterior process of the talus or of the sustentaculum tali may be fixed in a second step after making the diagnosis with postoperative CT via a posterior or medial approach, respectively.[32,33]

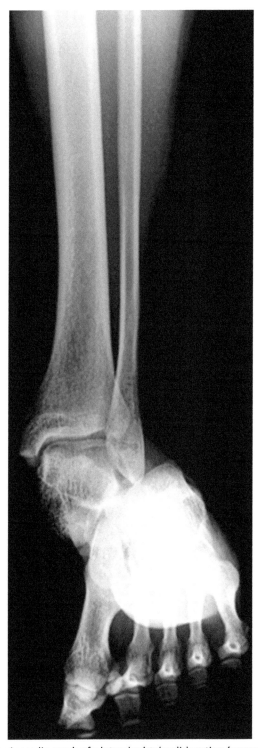

Fig. 2. Anteroposterior radiograph of a lateral subtalar dislocation (same patient as in **Fig. 1**).

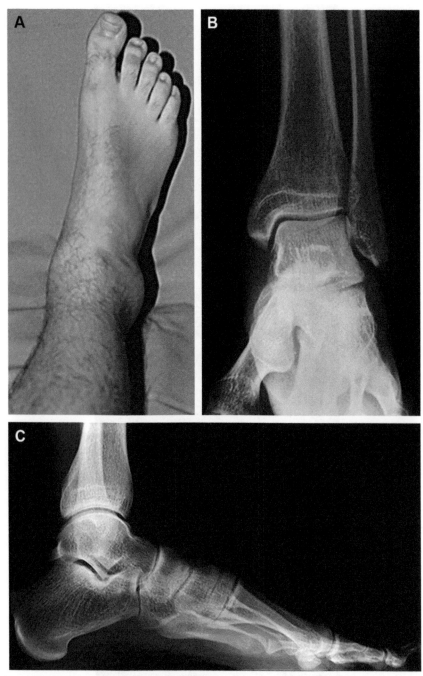

Fig. 3. (*A*) Clinical appearance and (*B*) radiographic image after closed reduction of a lateral subtalar dislocation. (*C*) The standing radiograph at 2 years shows no signs of instability or posttraumatic arthritis (same patient as in **Figs. 1** and **2**).

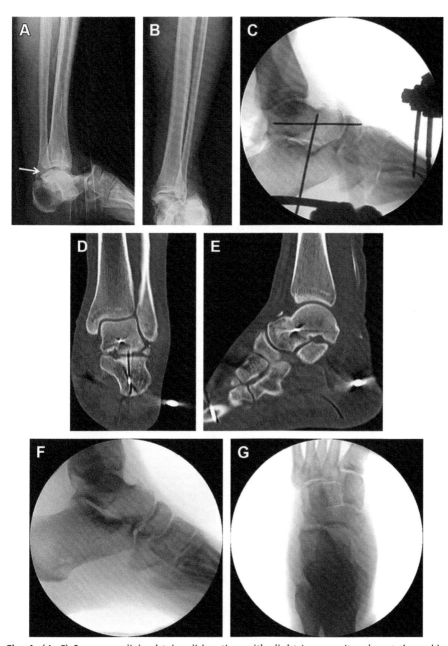

Fig. 4. (*A, B*) Severe medial subtalar dislocation with slight incongruity, also at the ankle joint (*arrow*). This case supports the theory that the total talar dislocation is a "second stage" of a subtalar dislocation. (*C*) Treatment consists of closed reduction and subsequent K-wire transfixation supplemented by external fixation because of severe instability. (*D, E*) Postreduction CT reveals a lateral talar process fracture that is treated with excision of the fragment and a capsular avulsion at the talonavicular joint. (*F, G*) The K-wires are removed after 4 weeks. At that time the subtalar joint appears clinically stable.

Anterior and posterior subtalar dislocations are reduced with axial traction to the affected foot with the knee flexed. In posterior dislocations, the forefoot is plantar-flexed to disengage the navicular from the undersurface of the talar neck and head. Then, the forefoot is brought into dorsiflexion while the heel is pulled distally. For anterior dislocations, longitudinal traction of the foot is followed by posterior (proximal) translation of the foot and axial traction on the heel.

Between 20% and 25% of all subtalar dislocations are open with lateral dislocations being affected more often than medial dislocations.[7,9] Open reduction is accompanied by copious lavage and wound debridement. With extensile soft tissue trauma, additional tibiometatarsal external fixation may assist with soft tissue consolidation (**Fig. 5**). If the wound cannot be closed without tension, artificial skin substitutes are used as a temporary cover followed by secondary suture. Rarely, a pedicled or free flap will be needed for definite wound coverage.

After successful reduction, the foot is immobilized in a cast for 6 weeks. Temporary K-wire transfixation of the subtalar joint is reserved for rare cases of marked instability after initial reduction. K-wires are removed after 3 to 4 weeks (see **Fig. 4**).

RESULTS AND COMPLICATIONS

Avascular necrosis (AVN) of the talus is a specific complication both after fractures and dislocations. Talar AVN has been noted after both medial and lateral subtalar

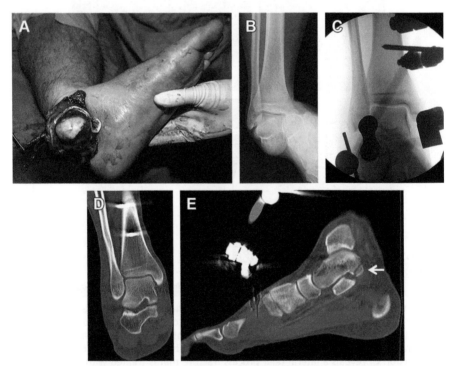

Fig. 5. (A) Open lateral subtalar dislocation. Anteroposterior radiographic image before (B) and after (C) open debridement, reduction, and external fixation. (D, E) Postreduction CT reveals an undisplaced posterior process fracture of the talus (arrow) that is treated nonoperatively.

dislocations. The reported rates range between 0% and 10% for closed disloca-tions and up to 50% for open dislocations.[7,22] In contrast with talar fractures,[34] aggressive management with early reduction and stable fixation if necessary helped to reduce these rates to about 10% in more recent studies.[35] Partial AVN of the talus without collapse of the talar dome does not require prolonged offload-ing or specific surgical treatment. Salvage of AVN with talar collapse consists of necrectomy, bone grafting, and fusion of the affected joint(s).[12] Neurovascular deficits may result from open injuries or incarceration of the deep posterior neuro-vascular bundle, especially with lateral dislocations. Tendon lacerations can occur after interposition, especially the tibialis posterior tendon, in lateral dislocations potentially leading to posttraumatic tendinitis and dysfunction. If partial or complete tears of the posterior tibial tendons are noted intraoperatively, primary repair is advised.[22]

Skin necrosis can be avoided with rapid reduction of the dislocation. Deep soft tissue and bone infections are only reported after open dislocations. Goldner and colleagues,[22] in a series of 15 open subtalar dislocations saw 1 case of osteomyelitis, 5 cases of AVN, and the need for secondary tibiotalar or subtalar fusion in 5 and 2 cases, respectively. Deep infections require repeat debridements and intravenous antibiotics. Resulting bony and soft tissue defects are reconstructed after eradication of infection.

Chronic ligamentous instability and recurrent subluxation after subtalar dislocations is rare and may be owing to early motion and immobilization of less than 4 weeks.[7] Treatment options include orthoses, muscle strengthening, proprioceptive training, ligamentoplasty, and fusion for gross instability with subsequent arthritis.[6] The reported rates of posttraumatic arthritis of the subtalar joint vary considerably between 40% and 89%; however, only about one-third of cases are symptomatic and warrant fusion.[8,20] Not surprisingly, patients with pure ligamentous injuries are less likely to develop arthritis than those with associated fractures.[25] For painful com-bined arthritis of the subtalar and talonavicular joint, some authors have advocated triple fusion.[22,36] Development of a complex regional pain syndrome type I is rare and may be associated with delayed reduction or incomplete analgesia.[37] Direct injury to the tibial nerve may lead to complex regional pain syndrome type II (causalgia) and may require surgical revision.

Prognosis after subtalar dislocation depends on the type of injury. Although purely ligamentous dislocations carry a good to excellent prognosis with early reduction,[38] less favorable results are seen with associated osseous and cartilaginous injuries (Fig. 6). Other negative prognostic factors include open subtalar dislocations and total talar dislocations. However, even for total talar dislocations, early replantation may result in favorable results.[39] In general, medial subtalar dislocations are associated with better outcomes than lateral subtalar dislocations.[40] This may reflect the more severe injury patterns with lateral dislocations because these are more often associ-ated with open injuries, fractures, and interposed soft tissues.[7,9] When looking at purely ligamentous dislocations only, Jungbluth and colleagues[38] found almost iden-tical outcomes after medial and lateral dislocations. Likewise, excellent functional results are reported in up to 100% after low-energy injuries; these numbers decrease to 15% in high-energy injuries.[22,23] In a recent literature review of 329 patients, Hoexum and Heetveld[9] found that functional results were reported to be good in 52%, fair in 25%, and poor in 23%. However, comparison between different studies is difficult because different outcome measurements have been used and many authors employed the American Orthopaedic Foot and Ankle Society score, which is not validated.

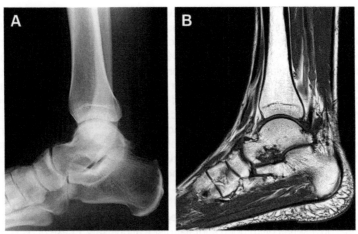

Fig. 6. (*A*) Two-year follow-up after open lateral subtalar dislocation without any signs of chronic instability (same patient as in **Fig. 5**). The patient complains about pain on exercise and when walking on uneven surfaces. (*B*) MRI reveals no signs of talar avascular necrosis or secondary dislocation of the posterior talar process but loss of cartilage at the subtalar joint as a sign of posttraumatic arthritis owing to the original energy of the injury.

SUMMARY

Purely ligamentous subtalar dislocations have an excellent prognosis with early reduction. If closed reduction is impossible because of locked dislocations or soft tissue interposition, open reduction is indicated. Complications such as AVN and posttraumatic arthritis are seen predominately after open dislocations, total talar dislocations, and associated fractures. Because more than 60% of subtalar dislocations are associated with talar process fractures or other bony injuries, a generous use of postreduction CT is recommended to ensure proper management of these injuries and avoid deleterious late sequelae of overlooked fractures at the hindfoot.

REFERENCES

1. DuFaurest P. Luxation du pied, en dehors, compliquee de l'issue de l'astragale a travers la capsule et les tegumens dechirees. J Med Chir Pharm 1811;22:348.
2. Broca P. Memoire sur les luxations sous-astragaliennes. Mem Soc Chir (Paris) 1953;3:566–656.
3. Malgaigne JF. Die Knochenbrüche und Verrenkungen. Stuttgart (Germany): Reiger; 1856.
4. Henke JW. Die Beweglichkeit des Fußes am Sprungbein. Z Rationelle Med 1855; 7:225.
5. Leitner B. Behandlungen und Behandlungsergebnisse von 42 frischen Fällen von Luxatio pedis sub talo im Unfallkrankenhaus Wien. Ergeb Chir Orthop 1952;37: 501–77.
6. Zwipp H. Chirurgie des Fußes. Wien (Austria); New York: Springer; 1994.
7. Zimmer TJ, Johnson KA. Subtalar dislocations. Clin Orthop 1989;238:190–4.
8. Heppenstall RB, Farahvar H, Balderston R, et al. Evaluation and management of subtalar dislocations. J Trauma 1980;20(6):494–7.
9. Hoexum F, Heetveld MJ. Subtalar dislocation: two cases requiring surgery and a literature review of the last 25 years. Arch Orthop Trauma Surg 2014;134(9):1237–49.

10. Bibbo C, Lin SS, Abidi N, et al. Missed and associated injuries after subtalar dislocation: the role of CT. Foot Ankle Int 2001;22(4):324–8.
11. Bohay DR, Manoli A 2nd. Occult fractures following subtalar joint injuries. Foot Ankle Int 1996;17(3):164–9.
12. Rammelt S, Winkler J, Grass R, et al. Reconstruction after talar fractures. Foot Ankle Clin 2006;11(1):61–84, viii.
13. Schmidt HM. Gestalt und Befestigung der Bandsysteme im Sinus und Canalis tarsi des Menschen. Acta Anat 1978;102:184–94.
14. Jotoku T, Kinoshita M, Okuda R, et al. Anatomy of ligamentous structures in the tarsal sinus and canal. Foot Ankle Int 2006;27(7):533–8.
15. Li SY, Hou ZD, Zhang P, et al. Ligament structures in the tarsal sinus and canal. Foot Ankle Int 2013;34(12):1729–36.
16. Weindel S, Schmidt R, Rammelt S, et al. Subtalar instability: a biomechanical cadaver study. Arch Orthop Trauma Surg 2010;130(3):313–9.
17. Panchani PN, Chappell TM, Moore GD, et al. Anatomic study of the deltoid ligament of the ankle. Foot Ankle Int 2014;35(9):916–21.
18. Schmidt HM, Grünwald E. Untersuchungen an den Bandsystemen der talocruralen und intertarsalen Gelenke des Menschen. Gegenbaurs Morphol Jahrb 1981; 127:792–831.
19. von Volkmann R. Ein Ligamentum "neglectum" pedis (Lig. calcaneonaviculare mediodorsale seu sustentaculonaviculare). Verh Anat Ges 1970;64:483–90.
20. Bibbo C, Anderson RB, Davis WH. Injury characteristics and the clinical outcome of subtalar dislocations: a clinical and radiographic analysis of 25 cases. Foot Ankle Int 2003;24(2):158–63.
21. Buckingham WW Jr, LeFlore I. Subtalar dislocation of the foot. J Trauma 1973; 13(9):753–65.
22. Goldner JL, Poletti SC, Gates HS 3rd, et al. Severe open subtalar dislocations. Long-term results. J Bone Joint Surg Am 1995;77(7):1075–9.
23. Grantham SA. Medical subtalar dislocation: five cases with a common etiology. J Trauma 1964;4:845–9.
24. Heck BE, Ebraheim NA, Jackson WT. Anatomical considerations of irreducible medial subtalar dislocation. Foot Ankle Int 1996;17(2):103–6.
25. Berkowitz MJ, Sanders R. Dislocations of the foot. In: Coughlin MJ, Saltzman CL, Anderson RB, editors. Mann's surgery of the foot and ankle. 9th edition. Philadelphia: Elsevier Saunders; 2013. p. 1905–72.
26. Baumgartner A, Huguier A. Les luxations sous-astragaliennes. Rev Chir 1907;36: 114–29.
27. Inokuchi S, Hashimoto T, Usami N. Anterior subtalar dislocation: case report. J Orthop Trauma 1997;11(3):235–7.
28. Inokuchi S, Hashimoto T, Usami N. Posterior subtalar dislocation. J Trauma 1997; 42(2):310–3.
29. Jarde O, Trinquier-Lautard JL, Mertl P, et al. Les luxations sous-astragaliennes. A propos de 35 cas. Rev Chir Orthop Reparatrice Appar Mot 1996;82(1):42–8.
30. Menetrey J, Fritschy D. Subtalar subluxation in ballet dancers. Am J Sports Med 1999;27(2):143–9.
31. Leitner B. Obstacles to reduction in subtalar dislocations. J Bone Joint Surg Am 1954;36(A:2):299–306.
32. Dürr C, Zwipp H, Rammelt S. Fractures of the sustentaculum tali. Oper Orthop Traumatol 2013;25(6):569–78.
33. Giuffrida AY, Lin SS, Abidi N, et al. Pseudo os trigonum sign: missed posteromedial talar facet fracture. Foot Ankle Int 2003;24(8):642–9.

34. Rammelt S, Zwipp H. Talar neck and body fractures. Injury 2009;40(2):120–35.
35. Milenkovic S, Mitkovic M, Bumbasirevic M. External fixation of open subtalar dislocation. Injury 2006;37(9):909–13.
36. Ruiz Valdivieso T, de Miguel Vielba JA, Hernandez Garcia C, et al. Subtalar dislocation. A study of nineteen cases. Int Orthop 1996;20(2):83–6.
37. Merchan EC. Subtalar dislocations: long-term follow-up of 39 cases. Injury 1992; 23(2):97–100.
38. Jungbluth P, Wild M, Hakimi M, et al. Isolated subtalar dislocation. J Bone Joint Surg Am 2010;92(4):890–4.
39. Assal M, Stern R. Total extrusion of the talus. A case report. J Bone Joint Surg Am 2004;86-A(12):2726–31.
40. de Palma L, Santucci A, Marinelli M, et al. Clinical outcome of closed isolated subtalar dislocations. Arch Orthop Trauma Surg 2008;128(6):593–8.

Subtalar Coalition in Pediatrics

Vincent S. Mosca, MD[a,b]

KEYWORDS

- Subtalar tarsal coalition • Talocalcaneal tarsal coalition
- Calcaneonavicular tarsal coalition • Tarsal coalition resection
- Calcaneal lengthening osteotomy

KEY POINTS

- Subtalar tarsal coalition is an autosomal dominant developmental maldeformation that affects between 2% and 13% of the population.
- The most common locations are between the calcaneus and navicular and between the talus and calcaneus.
- If prolonged attempts at nonoperative management do not relieve the pain, surgery is indicated.
- The exact surgical technique(s) should be based on the location of the pain, the size and histology of the coalition, the health of the other joints and facets, the degree of foot deformity, and the excursion of the heel cord.

DEFINITION

- Tarsal coalition is a fibrous, cartilaginous, or bony connection between 2 or more tarsal bones that results from a failure of differentiation and segmentation of primitive mesenchyme.
- It is a developmental maldeformation in that it is
  - Not present at birth (therefore, not congenital), although it is genetically programmed to develop
  - A synchondrosis/synostosis, which is in the category of malformation—failure to separate, and
  - Also a deformity, because most affected feet have valgus deformity of the hindfoot

No funding has been received in regard to the contents of this article and the author has no conflicts of interest to report.
[a] Pediatric Foot and Ankle Service, Seattle Children's Hospital, 4800 Sand Point Way, N.E, OA.9.120, Seattle, WA 98105, USA; [b] Department of Orthopaedics and Sports Medicine, University of Washington School of Medicine, 4333 Brooklyn Ave, N.E, Seattle, WA 98105, USA
E-mail address: vincent.mosca@seattlechildrens.org

Foot Ankle Clin N Am 20 (2015) 265–281
http://dx.doi.org/10.1016/j.fcl.2015.02.005
1083-7515/15/$ – see front matter © 2015 Elsevier Inc. All rights reserved.

EPIDEMIOLOGY

Tarsal coalition has been described in the archaeological remains of several civilizations since pre-Columbian times.[1] The association of the anatomic abnormality with the clinical syndrome of a painful flatfoot occurred 26 years after the introduction of radiographic imaging in 1895. In 1921, Slomann[2] linked the so-called peroneal spastic flatfoot with calcaneonavicular coalitions seen on radiographs. Almost 3 decades later, Harris and Beath[3,4] linked peroneal spastic flatfoot with talocalcaneal coalition. Tarsal coalition has also been linked with the infrequently occurring tibialis spastic varus, or cavovarus, foot since 1965.[5,6]

Some tarsal coalitions are associated with other congenital disorders, such as fibular hemimelia,[7] clubfoot,[8] Apert syndrome,[9] and Nievergelt-Pearlman syndrome. These tend to be extensive in regard to the number of tarsal bones involved and the percentage of involvement of the subtalar joint. The natural history and prognosis for these types, although not well studied, seem good.

More commonly, tarsal coalitions occur as isolated anomalies. The overall incidence of tarsal coalitions was proposed by Harris and Beath in 1948 as 2%, on the basis of routine physical examinations of Canadian Army enlistees.[3,4] On the basis of a cadaveric study by Phitzner in 1896, the rate of calcaneal navicular synostosis was found to be 2.9% and, if talocalcaneal coalitions are included, the incidence of tarsal coalition might reach 6%.[1,10] A radiographic study by Lysack and Fenton[11] documented a general prevalence of calcaneal navicular coalition of 5.6%, which was significantly greater than previously reported. And a recent cadaver study by Ruhli and colleagues[12] found the incidence of tarsal coalitions to be 13%.

The most common sites of coalition are in the middle facet of the talocalcaneal joint and between the anterior process of the calcaneus and the navicular.

- Talocalcaneal and calcaneonavicular coalitions occur with approximately equal frequency.[13]
  - Together, they account for approximately 90% of all coalitions.[13]
  - They coexist in a small percentage of feet.[14]
  - They are bilateral in 50% to 60% of cases.[15,16]
- Talonavicular, calcaneocuboid, naviculocuneiform, and cubonavicular coalitions are uncommon.[13]
- The true incidence of tarsal coalition, as well as the relative frequency of affected joints and the frequency of bilaterality, is not known, because most affected individuals are asymptomatic and go uncounted.

ETIOLOGY

Wray and Herndon[17] suggested an autosomal dominant pattern of inheritance with variable penetrance based on a single-family study. Leonard[18] confirmed an autosomal dominant pattern with almost full penetrance in a study of 31 index patients and 98 first-degree relatives. Tarsal coalitions have been found in monozygotic twins.[19]

CLINICAL FEATURES

- Progressive flattening of the longitudinal arch with valgus deformity of the hindfoot generally predates symptoms but is rarely the presenting complaint.
- The insidious onset of vague and aching pain in a child between the ages of 8 and 16 years is characteristic.

- ○ Pain may be located
  - ■ At the site of the coalition
    - • Only if it is still a synchondrosis; there can be no pain at a synostosis
  - ■ At the adjacent joints — Chopart joint (talonavicular and calcaneocuboid) and the ankle joint
    - • Due to stress transfer
  - ■ Under the flattened medial midfoot and/or in the sinus tarsi
    - • Due to the deformity, as occurs in flexible flatfoot with a short tendo-Achilles
- • The pain is usually aggravated by activity and relieved by rest.
- • Occasionally, children report recurrent ankle sprains.
- • There is often tenderness at the site of the coalition and there may be tenderness on the dorsal aspect of the talonavicular joint.
- • The flatfoot deformity has been variously described as rigid and peroneal spastic.
  - ○ Rigidity refers to restriction of subtalar joint motion, which can be assessed in several ways.
    - ■ When assessing subtalar motion, it is important to isolate and manipulate the subtalar joint with the ankle joint held in neutral dorsiflexion, with care taken to ensure that the apparent subtalar joint motion is, in fact, occurring at that joint.
      - • The talonavicular and calcaneocuboid joints can develop hypermobility in some feet with long-established and solid subtalar coalitions and can give the impression of subtalar joint motion when none exists.
    - ■ In a typical foot with a talocalcaneal coalition, the subtalar joint does not invert and the arch does not elevate during toe standing (**Fig. 1**)[20] or with the Jack toe-raising test.[21]
    - ■ Feet with calcaneonavicular coalitions are generally less rigid and less flat than those with talocalcaneal coalitions, which makes inherent sense because the former type does not bridge cross the subtalar joint and the latter does.
  - ○ Peroneal spastic is a poorly defined term that refers to apparent involuntary contracture of the peroneal tendons that appear to tent the skin posterior to the lateral malleolus. It is seen most often in a rigid flatfoot without a tarsal coalition. The etiology of the rigidity and the peroneal spasm has not been elucidated.

RADIOGRAPHIC FEATURES

- • A calcaneonavicular coalition is best seen on an oblique radiograph of the foot (**Fig. 2**A).
  - ○ A cartilaginous coalition has the appearance of an articulation with somewhat undulating subchondral bone surfaces.
  - ○ An osseous coalition is obvious. Its presence is suggested on the standing lateral radiograph by an elongated process of the anterior calcaneus, called the anteater nose sign (see **Fig. 2**B).[22]
- • A talocalcaneal coalition is difficult to appreciate on any standard radiographic view but is suggested on the lateral view.
  - ○ There may be dorsal beaking on the head of the talus (**Fig. 3**), broadening and rounding of the lateral process of the talus, and narrowing of the posterior talocalcaneal facet joint.[16,23]
  - ○ The C-sign, a C-shaped line formed by the confluence of the subchondral bone of the talar dome (talus) with the posterior edge of the middle facet coalition (talus and calcaneus) and the subchondral bone of the sustentaculum tali (calcaneus), is a fairly reliable indicator of a talocalcaneal coalition (see **Fig. 3**).[24]

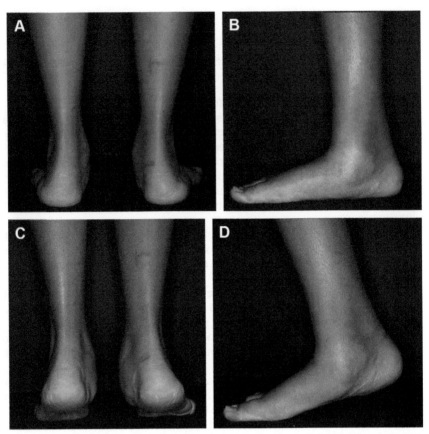

Fig. 1. (*A, B*) Rigid flatfoot. (*C, D*) The arch does not elevate, and the hindfoot valgus does not correct to varus during toe standing, because of immobility of the subtalar joint. (*From* Mosca VS. Flexible flatfoot and tarsal coalition. In: Richards B, editor. Orthopedic knowledge update: pediatrics. Rosemont (IL): American Academy of Orthopedic Surgeons; 1996. p. 211; with permission.)

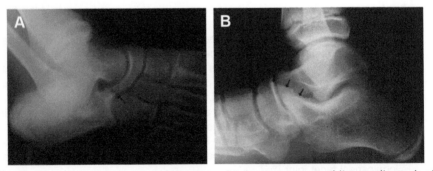

Fig. 2. (*A*) A calcaneonavicular coalition (*arrow*) is best seen on an oblique radiograph of the foot. (*B*) Lateral radiograph demonstrating the anteater nose sign (*arrows*), indicating a calcaneonavicular coalition. (*From* Mosca VS. The foot. In: Weinstein SL, Flynn JM, editors. Lovell and Winter's pediatric orthopedics. 7th edition. Philadelphia: Wolters Kluwer/Lippincott Williams & Wilkins; 2014. p. 1506. Fig. 29-132; with permission.)

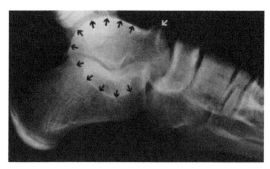

Fig. 3. A dorsal talar beak (*white arrow*) in a foot with a talocalcaneal coalition. This represents a traction spur, not degenerative arthritis. The C-sign of Lateur (*black arrows*) is a nonspecific indication of a talocalcaneal coalition. (*From* Mosca VS. The foot. In: Weinstein SL, Flynn JM, editors. Lovell and Winter's pediatric orthopedics. 7th edition. Philadelphia: Wolters Kluwer/Lippincott Williams & Wilkins; 2014. p. 1507. Fig. 29-133; with permission).

- It is not, however, pathognomonic. Taniguchi and colleagues[25] found the C-sign to have low sensitivity, meaning that the diagnosis of tarsal coalition is not negated by the absence of a C-sign. Brown and colleagues[26] found the C-sign specific for a flatfoot deformity but neither sensitive nor specific for the diagnosis of subtalar coalition. Liu and colleagues[27] found that an apparently absent middle facet was a more accurate sign in the diagnosis of a subtalar coalition than either talar beaking or the C-sign.
  - An anteroposterior radiograph of the ankle should also be obtained.
    - A ball-and-socket ankle may be seen in cases of longstanding tarsal coalition, particularly with the large coalitions seen in the nonidiopathic types.[7,8]
  - A talocalcaneal coalition can be seen on an axial, or Harris,[3,4] radiograph, but the best way to assess a coalition in this location is with a CT scan (**Fig. 4**).[28,29]
    - The thin-slice images should be obtained in the coronal, sagittal, and transverse planes with 3-D reconstruction of the images.
  - A CT scan should also be obtained prior to resection of a calcaneonavicular coalition for 2 reasons:
    - The first is to clearly define the variable pathoanatomy of the coalition that, in extensive cases, may extend further plantar-medially under the head of the talus than might be suggested by the plane radiographs.[30]
    - The second is to determine if there is a coexisting talocalcaneal coalition, a situation not uncommonly seen.[14]

OTHER IMAGING STUDIES

More recently, Emery and colleagues[31] showed that MRI was nearly as good as the gold standard CT imaging for assessing subtalar coalitions. Although MRI should not be the first-line study, it can be used to identify a symptomatic tarsal coalition that is still in the fibrous stage of differentiation if the plain radiographs and CT scan are nondiagnostic.[32] A bone scan can help identify the true cause of pain in a foot that has radiographic evidence of a tarsal coalition but an atypical history or pain pattern.[29] Published treatment algorithms are base on CT scan findings.

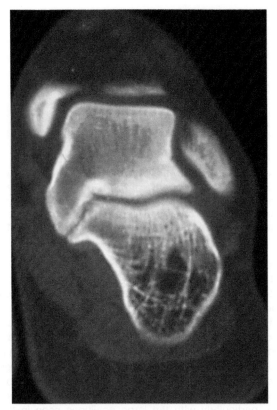

Fig. 4. Talocalcaneal coalitions are best seen on CT scans taken in the coronal plane. The middle facet is very narrow, irregular, and down-sloping. The posterior facet is more narrow than the ankle joint. And the calcaneus is in valgus alignment. (*From* Mosca VS. Flexible flatfoot and tarsal coalition. In: Richards B, editor. Orthopedic knowledge update: pediatrics. Rosemont (IL): American Academy of Orthopedic Surgeons; 1996. p. 211; with permission.)

OTHER DIAGNOSTIC STUDIES

Other causes for a rigid flatfoot include

- Juvenile rheumatoid arthritis
- Septic arthritis
- Osteomyelitis

A complete blood cell count with differential, estimated sedimentation rate, C-reactive protein, antinuclear antibody test, and rheumatoid factor may be warranted if evaluation fails to confirm a suspected tarsal coalition.

PATHOANATOMY

In genetically programmed individuals, a tarsal coalition begins as a syndesmosis with fibrous tissue between 2 bones of the foot that do not joint together in 87% to 98% of people. The fibrous tissue undergoes metaplasia to cartilage to become a synchondrosis and then to bone as a synostosis. This process occurs during late childhood and early to middle adolescence.[3,4,33,34]

Restriction of subtalar motion caused by a coalition blocks eversion of the subtalar complex that normally occurs during the early stance phase of gait. A component of eversion is dorsiflexion of the acetabulum pedis (anterior calcaneus, spring ligament, and navicular) that occurs as it laterally rotates and glides around the head of the talus. When rotation and gliding are eliminated by the coalition, the dorsiflexion force is concentrated at the talonavicular and calcaneocuboid joints.[35] They are converted to hinge joints that widen/distract inferiorly and narrow/compress superiorly. The dorsal proximal edge of the navicular impinges on and overrides the head of the talus. This overriding causes elevation of the dorsal talonavicular ligament and periosteum on the dorsal neck of the talus. The osseus repair of this periosteal elevation leads to the talar beaking that is visible on lateral radiographs of the foot (see **Fig. 3**). The reason for progressive flattening of the longitudinal arch, which develops in most feet with tarsal coalitions, is not established.

The site or sites of pain vary from one individual to another. The cause of the pain is also variable and not necessarily known[3,4,13] but has been attributed to ligament sprain, peroneal muscle spasm, sinus tarsi impingement and irritation, subtalar joint irritation, fracture through the synchondrosis, and stress transfer to adjacent mobile joints with the development of degenerative arthrosis.[36] Pain can also be related to the flatfoot deformity itself that is often associated with a short tendo-Achilles.

NATURAL HISTORY

According to Leonard,[18] only approximately 25% of individuals with tarsal coalitions become symptomatic. The onset of pain usually coincides with metaplasia of the coalition from cartilage to bone but may occur earlier in its evolution. This generally occurs between 8 and 12 years for children with calcaneonavicular coalitions and between 12 and 16 years for those with talocalcaneal coalitions. Metaplasia of the coalition also, most often, coincides with the development of progressive valgus deformity of the hindfoot, flattening of the longitudinal arch, and restriction of subtalar motion. All these findings are more severe in feet with talocalcaneal coalitions.[16,33]

TREATMENT

- Treatment is indicated only for persistently painful tarsal coalitions,[3,4,15,16] because there is no published evidence that painless tarsal coalitions cause disability.
- There is also no evidence that resection of painless, incidentally identified tarsal coalitions leads to better outcomes than the natural history of the condition.
- It is not clear what causes some to become painful, but inflammation clearly underlies the pain, wherever it is located.
- Attempts should be made to relieve symptoms by nonoperative means, which may include activity modification, nonsteroidal anti-inflammatory drugs, over-the-counter shoe inserts, and immobilization in a cast-type walking boot or a below-the-knee walking cast.
  - Pain is generally relieved completely within 24 to 48 hours of cast/boot application.
  - Approximately 30% of patients remain pain-free after cast removal 6 weeks later.[33]
  - An over-the-counter shoe insert may help to maintain pain relief.
- The over-the-counter inexpensive shoe insert must not have a firm or hard arch elevation.

- ○ It must be flat and merely provide additional cushioning for the plantar aspect of the foot. These feet lack subtalar motion. The subtalar joint cannot be inverted by any means, passive or active. A firm or hard arch support increases pressure under the rigidly plantar flexed talar head and increases pain at that site.
- Surgery is indicated for those feet with persistent or recurrent disabling pain despite prolonged attempts at nonoperative management.
  - ○ The goal of treatment is to relief pain, not necessarily to eliminate the coalition or re-establish the longitudinal arch, although the latter outcomes may be part of the treatment.
  - ○ Surgical options include
    - ▪ Resection of the coalition
    - ▪ Deformity correction with an osteotomy
    - ▪ A combination of resection and deformity correction
    - ▪ Arthrodesis
- Resection of calcaneonavicular coalitions was first reported by Badgley[37] in 1927.
  - ○ Interposition of the extensor digitorum brevis (EDB) was added to the resection procedure and reported by Cowell[38] in 1970. Mubarak and colleagues,[39] in 2009, reported the advantages of using a free fat graft, rather than the EDB, because that interposition material led to lower reossification and reoperation rates and improved cosmesis. The combined procedure of resection and soft tissue interposition, compared with resection alone, has been shown to decrease the incidence of recurrence and to increase the incidence of long-term pain relief.[38–41]
- Resection of a calcaneonavicular coalition with muscle or fat interposition (**Fig. 5**) is indicated
  - ○ In patients younger than 16 years of age who have a cartilaginous bar
  - ○ With no other coalitions present
  - ○ And no degenerative arthrosis
  - ○ And who have persistent disabling pain despite prolonged attempts at nonoperative treatment[39,40]
    - ▪ The upper and lower age limits, as well as the influence of the coalition tissue type and the coexistence of other coalitions, have not been scientifically established.
- Prior to resection of a calcaneonavicular coalition
  - ○ It should be ensured that a second coalition is not present by analysis of a CT scan of the hindfoot.
  - ○ The absence of degenerative changes in the talonavicular joint and calcaneocuboid joint should be ensured. Significant degenerative arthritis is a contraindication to surgical excision.
  - ○ The 3-D anatomy of the coalition must be known.
    - ▪ Cooperman and colleagues[42] demonstrated significant variation in the extent of the fusion of the anterior aspect of the calcaneus with the navicular. In their analysis of 30 specimens, the anterior facet of the subtalar joint was totally spared in 8. The anterior facet was partially replaced in 7 of 30 specimens and completely replaced in 15. This variation in the anterior portion of the subtalar joint, related to calcaneonavicular coalitions, may result in some variation in outcome and certainly relates to the extent and depth of the resection required to adequately treat this problem. Failure to resolve symptoms with excision is often related to inadequate resection.[30] Upasani and colleagues[30] used CT scan analysis to show that

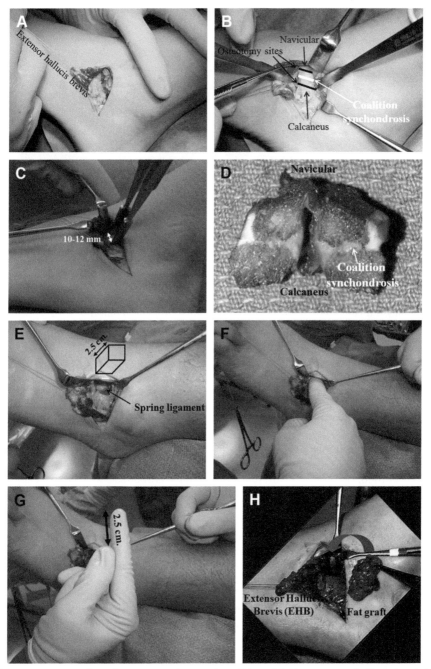

Fig. 5. Resection of a calcaneonavicular tarsal coalition. (*A*) The extensor hallucis brevis is elevated from the sinus tarsi and reflected anteriorly. (*B*) The synchondrosis and adjacent portions of the calcaneus and the navicular are exposed. (*C*) Ten-mm osteotomes are positioned 10–12 mm apart and parallel to each other for the osteotomies. (*D*) A resected coalition has been bisected to reveal the pathoanatomy. (*E*) The 3-D rectangle-shaped resection cavity is visualized with the spring ligament exposed at its base. (*F*) The resection cavity is large enough to accept the surgeon's index finger. (*G*) The cavity is 2.5 cm deep. (*H*) After the osteotomy surfaces are coated with bone wax, a large free fat graft is inserted to completely fill the cavity. The EHB is pulled over the fat graft and reattached to its origin in the sinus tarsi.

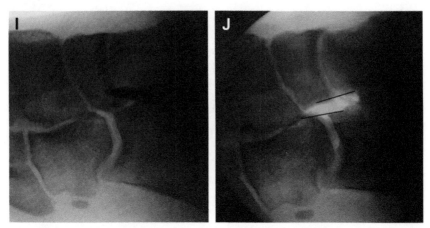

Fig. 5. (*continued*). Resection of a calcaneonavicular tarsal coalition. (*I*) Preresection obli-que intraoperative fluoroscopy image with osteotome in place. (*J*) Postresection oblique im-age. The navicular osteotomy is made in line with the head/neck of the talus. The calcaneus osteotomy is made in line with cuboid/lateral cuneiform joint. (*From* Mosca VS. Principles and management of pediatric foot and ankle deformities and malformations. Philadelphia: Wolters Kluwer/Lippincott Williams & Wilkins; 2014. p. 201–2. Fig. 8-4; with permission.)

  calcaneonavicular coalitions are usually 25 mm deep (from dorsolateral to plantar-medial) and wrap under the head of the talus. They suggested using a preoperative CT scan for surgical planning.
- The role of surgical resection of a talocalcaneal coalition is less clear.
  - This coalition is located on the tension side of the valgus deformity of the hind-foot, and further progressive flattening of the arch has been reported after resection.
  - In 1948, Harris and Beath[4] reported that triple arthrodesis was the most appro-priate treatment of persistently symptomatic talocalcaneal coalitions, although they thought that resection was appropriate for calcaneonavicular bars.
- Resection of talocalcaneal coalitions became popular in the 1980s based on a frequently quoted, but unsubstantiated, statement in the literature that a talocal-caneal coalition could be successfully resected as long as it occupied less than half the width of the subtalar joint surface.[43] Investigations have recently attemp-ted to validate that statement.
  - In 1994, Wilde and colleagues[44] reported unsatisfactory results of resection in feet in which the ratio of the surface area of the coalition to the surface area of the posterior facet was greater than 50% (as determined by CT mapping of the entire joint). There was excessive valgus deformity of the hindfoot in all of these feet, measured on the coronal CT images as greater than 16°. Many of the feet with poor outcomes also had narrowing of the posterior facet and impingement of the lateral process of the talus on the calcaneus. The independent influence of the size of the coalition was not established by this or any study to date.
  - Luhmann and Schoenecker[45] reported that there were good postoperative re-sults after resection in feet with valgus deformities of less than 21° and with middle facet involvement of more than 50%. Valgus deformity in excess of 21°, however, required postoperative bracing and had compromised results.
  - The Wilde and colleagues[44] criteria remain the most objective criteria for deter-mining the resectability of a talocalcaneal tarsal coalition (**Fig. 6**).

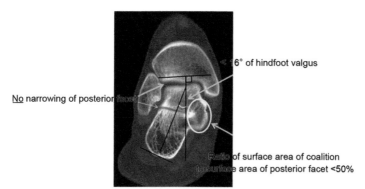

6° of hindfoot valgus

No narrowing of posterior facet

Ratio of surface area of coalition to surface area of posterior facet <50%

Fig. 6. Coronal slice CT scan image shows the 3 criteria for resectability of a talocalcaneal tarsal coalition according to Wilde and colleagues: (1) the ratio of the surface area of the coalition of the middle facet (*yellow oval*) to the surface area of the posterior facet should be less than 50%; (2) there should be no narrowing of the posterior facet (*thin green arrow*) compared with the cartilage height of the ankle joint (*thick green arrow*); and (3) there should be less than 16° of hindfoot valgus measured between the axis of the calcaneus and the line perpendicular to the ankle joint (*yellow arc*). None of the 3 criteria for resectability is met on this image. (*From* Mosca VS. Principles and management of pediatric foot and ankle deformities and malformations. Philadelphia: Wolters Kluwer/Lippincott Williams & Wilkins; 2014. p. 104. Fig. 5-49; with permission).

- Degenerative arthrosis in the subtalar joint complex (including the talonavicular and calcaneocuboid joints) associated with either a talocalcaneal or calcaneonavicular coalition is considered a contraindication to resection, but that diagnosis is difficult to establish.
  - Historically, the presence of a dorsal talar beak was considered evidence of degenerative arthrosis. That theory was replaced with the belief that the beak represents a traction spur, because it recedes with successful resection of the coalition. Its presence is, therefore, not a contraindication to resection.[43,44,46,47]
- Successful resection and interposition grafting of talocalcaneal coalitions (**Fig. 7**) have been reported in up to 89% of cases at 10 years' follow-up,[48] although most published and unpublished studies have documented a lower success rate at even shorter follow-up.[44,46,49]
  - The poor results have been attributed to poor indications.
  - Interposition can be with fat[43,50] or a split portion of the flexor hallucis longus tendon.[49]
- Triple arthrodesis has been recommended by some investigators[4,36,43,44] for
  - Documented degenerative arthrosis in the subtalar joint complex (particularly in adults)
  - Persistent or recurrent pain and/or deformity following resection of a coalition
  - Large irresectable coalitions with severe valgus deformity of the hindfoot
    - The known poor long-term outcomes of triple arthrodesis,[51–55] however, make this an undesirable option, particularly for children and adolescents.
- Osteotomies performed to improve alignment of the foot, with or without resection of the coalition, are alternatives to arthrodesis.[56–65]
  - In a foot with a talocalcaneal tarsal coalition and severe hindfoot valgus deformity, the pain is often related to the deformity itself and not the coalition.[65]

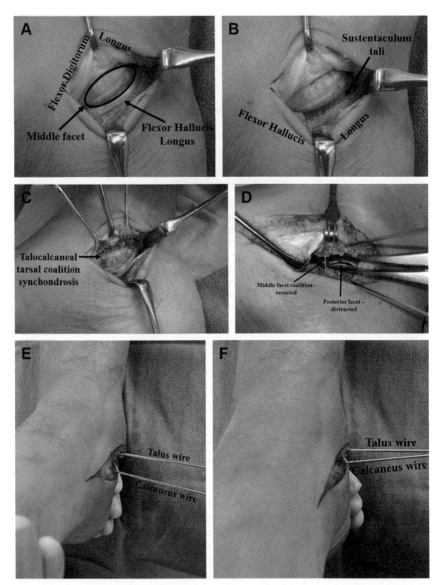

Fig. 7. Resection of a talocalcaneal tarsal coalition. (*A*) The flexor digitorum longus is retracted dorsally to expose the middle facet, although it might be easier to retract it plantarward in some feet. (*B*) The flexor hallucis longus is retracted plantarward from the sustentaculum tali. (*C*) The periosteum is sharply elevated from the medial surfaces of the talus and calcaneus at the middle facet. The synchondrosis is exposed. (*D*) The middle facet coalition has been resected. The posterior facet is visualized at the base of the resection cavity. An AO smooth-toothed laminar spreader in the resected middle facet cavity has been used to distract the posterior facet to ensure that there are no remaining bony or cartilaginous connections between the talus and calcaneus. (*E*) Steinmann pins are inserted in the talus and calcaneus from medial to lateral before resection of the coalition. There is no motion between them with attempted inversion and eversion of the subtalar joint. (*F*) After resection, convergence and divergence of the pins confirms restoration of subtalar motion.

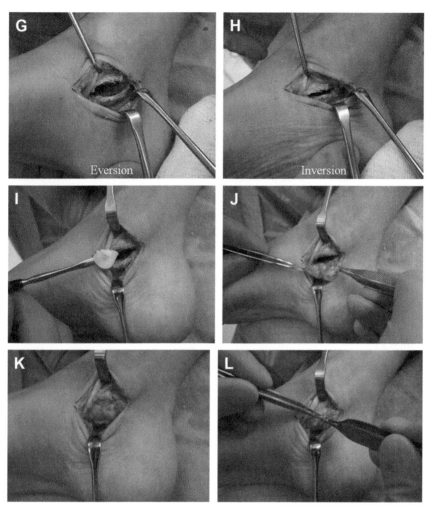

Fig. 7. (*continued*). Resection of a talocalcaneal tarsal coalition. (*G, H*) Direct visualization of the resection cavity during eversion and inversion of the subtalar joint, with widening and narrowing of the resection cavity, further confirms complete resection of the coalition. (*I*) Bone wax is applied to the resected bone surfaces. (*J*) A large free fat graft is inserted. (*K*) The fat graft completely fills the cavity. (*L*) The periosteum is repaired over the fat. The flexor retinaculum is subsequently repaired over the graft and the flexor tendons. (*From* Mosca VS. Principles and management of pediatric foot and ankle deformities and malformations. Philadelphia: Wolters Kluwer/Lippincott Williams & Wilkins; 2014. p. 203–4, Fig. 8-5; with permission.)

- There is pain, tenderness, and callus formation under the head of the plantar flexed talus, essentially identical to the signs and symptoms found in a flexible flatfoot with tight Achilles tendon.
- These feet often have large osseous talocalcaneal coalitions along with contracture of the gastrocnemius or the entire triceps surae.[65]
  ○ The posterior calcaneus medial displacement osteotomy, with or without a medial closing wedge, can be considered,[56–58] although those procedures

do not realign the talonavicular joint or correct the rotational deformity of the subtalar joint.

o The calcaneal lengthening osteotomy, conceptualized by Evans[59] and elaborated by Mosca,[60–64] has been shown by Mosca and Bevan[65] to correct all components of the everted valgus deformity of the hindfoot and relieve symptoms, even in feet with large, unresected, and unresectable middle facet osseous coalitions.

■ This osteotomy should be considered for
  • The rigid flatfoot with severe valgus deformity of the hindfoot and contracture of the Achilles tendon
  • Pain under the head of the talus (plantar-medial midfoot)
  • And little-to-no degenerative arthrosis of the talonavicular and calcaneocuboid joints

■ According to Mosca and Bevan,[65] the calcaneal lengthening osteotomy can be performed
  • As an isolated procedure if the pain is due to the deformity and the coalition is unresectable based on the criteria of Wilde and colleagues[44] (ie, large middle facet coalition and narrow posterior facet)
  • With concurrent or staged resection of the coalition and interposition fat grafting in a foot with severe valgus deformity and a resectable coalition

REFERENCES

1. Heiple KG, Lovejoy CO. The antiquity of tarsal coalition. Bilateral deformity in a Pre-Columbian Indian skeleton. J Bone Joint Surg Am 1969;51:979–83.
2. Slomann W. On coalitio calcaneo-navicularis. J Orthop Surg 1921;3:586.
3. Harris RI, Beath T. Army foot survey: an investigation of foot ailments in Canadian soldiers. National Research Council of Canada; 1947.
4. Harris R, Beath T. Etiology of peroneal spastic flatfoot. J Bone Joint Surg Br 1948; 30:624.
5. Simmons E. Tibialis spastic varus foot with tarsal coalition. J Bone Joint Surg Br 1965;47:533–6.
6. Stuecker R, Bennett J. Tarsal coalition presenting as a pes cavo-varus deformity: report of three cases and review of the literature. Foot Ankle 1993;14:540–4.
7. Grogan DP, Holt GR, Ogden JA. Talocalcaneal coalition in patients who have fibular hemimelia or proximal femoral focal deficiency. A comparison of the radiographic and pathological findings. J Bone Joint Surg Am 1994;76:1363–70.
8. Spero CR, Simon GS, Tornetta P III. Clubfeet and tarsal coalition. J Pediatr Orthop 1994;14:372–6.
9. Mah J, Kasser J, Upton J. The foot in Apert syndrome. Clin Plast Surg 1991;18: 391–7.
10. Herschel H, Ronnen JR. The occurrence of calcaneonavicular synosteosis in pes valgus contractus. J Bone Joint Surg Am 1950;32A:280–2.
11. Lysack JT, Fenton PV. Variations in calcaneonavicular morphology demonstrated with radiography. Radiology 2004;230:493–7.
12. Ruhli FJ, Solomon LB, Henneberg M. High prevalence of tarsal coalitions and tarsal joint variants in a recent cadaver sample and its possible significance. Clin Anat 2003;16(5):411–5.
13. Stormont DM, Peterson HA. The relative incidence of tarsal coalition. Clin Orthop Relat Res 1983;181:28–36.

14. Clarke DM. Multiple tarsal coalitions in the same foot. J Pediatr Orthop 1997;17: 777–80.
15. Cowell H. Tarsal coalition–review and update. Instr Course Lect 1982;31:264–71.
16. Drennan J. Tarsal coalitions. Instr Course Lect 1996;45:323–9.
17. Wray J, Herndon C. Hereditary transmission of congenital coalition of the calcaneus to the navicular. J Bone Joint Surg Am 1963;45:365.
18. Leonard MA. The inheritance of tarsal coalition and its relationship to spastic flat foot. J Bone Joint Surg Br 1974;56B:520–6.
19. Glessner JR Jr, Davis GL. Bilateral calcaneonavicular coalition occurring in twin boys. A case report. Clin Orthop Relat Res 1966;47:173–6.
20. Mosca VS. Flexible flatfoot and tarsal coalition. In: Richards B, editor. Orthopaedic knowledge update: pediatrics. Rosemont (IL): American Academy of Orthopaedic Surgeons; 1996. p. 211.
21. Jack EA. Naviculo-cuneiform fusion in the treatment of flat foot. J Bone Joint Surg Br 1953;35B:75–82.
22. Oestreich AE, Mize WA, Crawford AH, et al. The "anteater nose": a direct sign of calcaneonavicular coalition on the lateral radiograph. J Pediatr Orthop 1987;7:709–11.
23. Conway JJ, Cowell HR. Tarsal coalition: clinical significance and roentgenographic demonstration. Radiology 1969;92:799–811.
24. Lateur LM, Hoe LR, Ghillewe KV, et al. Subtalar coalition: diagnosis with the C sign on lateral radiographs of the ankle. Radiology 1994;193:847–51.
25. Taniguchi A, Tanaka Y, Kadono K, et al. C sign for diagnosis of talocalcaneal coalition. Radiology 2003;228:501–5.
26. Brown RR, Rosenberg ZS, Thornhill BA. The C sign: more specific for flatfoot deformity than subtalar coalition. Skeletal Radiol 2001;30:84–7.
27. Liu PT, Roberts CC, Chivers FS, et al. "Absent middle facet": a sign on unenhanced radiography of subtalar joint coalition. AJR Am J Roentgenol 2003;181: 1565–72.
28. Herzenberg JE, Goldner JL, Martinez S, et al. Computerized tomography of talocalcaneal tarsal coalition: a clinical and anatomic study. Foot Ankle 1986;6: 273–88.
29. Deutsch AL, Resnick D, Campbell G. Computed tomography and bone scintigraphy in the evaluation of tarsal coalition. Radiology 1982;144:137–40.
30. Upasani VV, Chambers RC, Mubarak SJ. Analysis of calcaneonavicular coalitions using multi-planar 3-dimensional computed tomography. J Child Orthop 2008;2: 301–7.
31. Emery KH, Bisset GS III, Johnson ND, et al. Tarsal coalition: a blinded comparison of MRI and CT. Pediatr Radiol 1998;28:612–6.
32. Wechsler RJ, Schweitzer ME, Deely DM, et al. Tarsal coalition: depiction and characterization with CT and MR imaging. Radiology 1994;193:447–52.
33. Jayakumar S, Cowell HR. Rigid flatfoot. Clin Orthop Relat Res 1977;122:77–84.
34. Kumai T, Takakura Y, Akiyama K, et al. Histopathologic study of nonosseous tarsal coalition. Foot Ankle Int 1998;19:525–31.
35. Outland T, Murphy ID. The pathomechanics of peroneal spastic flat foot. Clin Orthop Relat Res 1960;16:64–73.
36. Mosier KM, Asher M. Tarsal coalitions and peroneal spastic flat foot. A review. J Bone Joint Surg Am 1984;66:976–84.
37. Badgley C. Coalition of the calcaneus and the navicular. Arch Surg 1927;15:75.
38. Cowell H. Extensor brevis arthroplasty. J Bone Joint Surg Am 1970;82:820.
39. Mubarak SJ, Patel PN, Upasani VV, et al. Calcaneonavicular coalition: treatment by excision and fat graft. J Pediatr Orthop 2009;29:418–26.

40. Gonzalez P, Kumar SJ. Calcaneonavicular coalition treated by resection and interposition of the extensor digitorum brevis muscle. J Bone Joint Surg Am 1990;72:71–7.
41. Moyes ST, Crawfurd EJ, Aichroth PM. The interposition of extensor digitorum brevis in the resection of calcaneonavicular bars. J Pediatr Orthop 1994;14: 387–8.
42. Cooperman DR, Janke BE, Gilmore A, et al. A three-dimensional study of calcaneonavicular tarsal coalitions. J Pediatr Orthop 2001;21:648–51.
43. Scranton PE Jr. Treatment of symptomatic talocalcaneal coalition. J Bone Joint Surg Am 1987;69:533–9.
44. Wilde PH, Torode IP, Dickens DR, et al. Resection for symptomatic talocalcaneal coalition. J Bone Joint Surg Br 1994;76:797–801.
45. Luhmann SJ, Schoenecker PL. Symptomatic talocalcaneal coalition resection: indications and results. J Pediatr Orthop 1998;18:748–54.
46. Swiontkowski MF, Scranton PE, Hansen S. Tarsal coalitions: long-term results of surgical treatment. J Pediatr Orthop 1983;3:287–92.
47. Takakura Y, Sugimoto K, Tanaka Y, et al. Symptomatic talocalcaneal coalition. Its clinical significance and treatment. Clin Orthop Relat Res 1991;(269):249–56.
48. McCormack T, Olney B, Asher M. Talocalcaneal coalition resection: a 10-year follow-up. J Pediatr Orthop 1997;17:13–5.
49. Kumar SJ, Guille JT, Lee MS, et al. Osseous and non-osseous coalition of the middle facet of the talocalcaneal joint. J Bone Joint Surg Am 1992;74:529–35.
50. Olney BW, Asher MA. Excision of symptomatic coalition of the middle facet of the talocalcaneal joint. J Bone Joint Surg Am 1987;69:539–44.
51. Drew AJ. The late results of arthrodesis of the foot. J Bone Joint Surg Br 1951;33: 496–502.
52. Adelaar RS, Dannelly EA, Meunier PA, et al. A long-term study of triple arthrodesis in children. Orthop Clin North Am 1976;7:895–908.
53. Southwell RB, Sherman FC. Triple arthrodesis: a long-term study with force plate analysis. Foot Ankle 1981;2:15–24.
54. Angus PD, Cowell HR. Triple arthrodesis. A critical long-term review. J Bone Joint Surg Br 1986;68:260–5.
55. Saltzman CL, Fehrle MJ, Cooper RR, et al. Triple arthrodesis: twenty-five and forty-four year average follow-up of the same patients. J Bone Joint Surg Am 1999;81:1391–402.
56. Koutsogiannis E. Treatment of mobile flat foot by displacement osteotomy of the calcaneus. J Bone Joint Surg Br 1971;53:96–100.
57. Dwyer FC. President's address. Causes, significance and treatment of stiffness of the subtaloid joint. Proc R Soc Med 1976;69(2):97–102.
58. Cain TJ, Hyman S. Peroneal spastic flat foot. Its treatment by osteotomy of the os calcis. J Bone Joint Surg Br 1978;60:527–9.
59. Evans D. Calcaneo-valgus deformity. J Bone Joint Surg Br 1975;57:270–8.
60. Mosca VS. Calcaneal lengthening for valgus deformity of the hindfoot. Results in children who had severe, symptomatic flatfoot and skewfoot. J Bone Joint Surg Am 1995;77:500–12.
61. Mosca VS. Calcaneal lengthening osteotomy for valgus deformity of the hindfoot. In: Skaggs DL, Tolo VT, editors. Master techniques in orthopaedic surgery: pediatrics. Philadelphia: Lippincott Williams & Wilkins; 2008. p. 263–76.
62. Mosca VS. Calcaneal lengthening osteotomy for the treatment of hindfoot valgus deformity. In: Wiesel S, editor. Operative techniques in orthopaedic surgery. Philadelphia: Lippincott Williams & Wilkins; 2010. p. 1608–18.

63. Mosca VS. The foot. In: Weinstein SL, Flynn JM, editors. Lovell and Winter's pediatric orthopedics. 7th edition. Philadelphia: Wolters Kluwer/Lippincott Williams & Wilkins; 2014. p. 1425–562.

64. Mosca VS. Principles and management of pediatric foot and ankle deformities and malformations. Philadelphia: Wolters Kluwer/Lippincott Williams & Wilkins; 2014.

65. Mosca VS, Bevan WP. Talocalcaneal tarsal coalitions and the calcaneal lengthening osteotomy: the role of deformity correction. J Bone Joint Surg Am 2012; 94:1584–94.

Subtalar Coalitions in the Adult

James F. Flynn, MD, Dane K. Wukich, MD*, Stephen F. Conti, MD,
Carl T. Hasselman, MD, Macalus V. Hogan, MD, Alex J. Kline, MD

KEYWORDS

- Subtalar • Coalition • Adults • Flatfeet • Hindfoot • Valgus

KEY POINTS

- Subtalar coalition in adults may present with a painful pes planovalgus deformity.
- Nonsurgical management has varying degrees of success and surgery is often required.
- In the presence of arthritic change, arthrodesis should be offered to the patient, which may be done arthroscopically if isolated to the subtalar joint, if alignment is appropriate, and if the surgeon has the requisite technical skills.

INTRODUCTION

A tarsal coalition is a bony or fibrous union of 2 or more tarsal bones. Its incidence has been reported as roughly 1% of the overall population, but may be significantly higher as many are asymptomatic or missed.[1–5] A computerized tomographic (CT) study on cadaveric feet suggested that subtalar coalitions may be present in as high as 12.7% of the population.[6] The most common tarsal coalitions occur between the calcaneus and the navicular (53%) or between the talus and the calcaneus, specifically at the middle facet of the subtalar joint (37%).[1,3,5,7]

The cause of a congenital tarsal coalition is a failure of the mesenchymal cells in the embryo to differentiate and segment. Coalitions are inherited in an autosomal-dominant pattern.[7–9] Rarely, and more in adults than adolescents, a coalition may be acquired from trauma, surgery, infection, arthritis, or neoplasia.[4,10]

Many of the studies on coalitions have focused on the pediatric/adolescent population, in which symptoms such as peroneal spastic flatfoot may present as the coalition begins to ossify.[11] In the adult population, many tarsal coalitions are

Dr C.T. Hasselman is a consultant for Arthrex and Arthrosurface and Dr D.K. Wukich is a consultant for Stryker and receives royalties from Arthrex. Dr S.F. Conti, Dr J.F. Flynn, Dr M.V. Hogan, and Dr A.J. Kline have nothing to disclose.
Orthopaedic Foot and Ankle Fellowship Program, University of Pittsburgh, Pittsburgh, PA, USA
* Corresponding author. UPMC Mercy Health Center, 1515 Locust Street, Suite 325, Pittsburgh, PA 15219.
E-mail address: wukichdk@upmc.edu

discovered incidentally while a patient is being evaluated for a different condition.[5] Varner and Michelson[12] retrospectively reviewed 27 adult patients with a coalition and found that two-thirds of these were discovered during workup for symptoms such as an ankle instability and sinus tarsi pain, whereas one-third of the adult patients were completely asymptomatic.[12] Rankin and Baker[13] reported that in 24 military recruits undergoing basic training, symptoms may initially present after stressful activity, but further inquiry revealed prior history of foot pain.[13] Other case reports have shown incidental discovery of a coalition during the workup for a talar body fracture[14] or cavovarus foot deformity.[15] Recently, a fracture of a subtalar coalition was discovered during a workup for an ankle sprain.[16]

EVALUATION

Although deep subtalar joint pain[3,5] may cause a patient with a talocalcaneal coalition to present for evaluation, other symptoms can be varied and nonspecific. These symptoms range from ankle instability and sinus tarsi pain[12] to slowly resolving pain after a seemingly innocuous foot or ankle injury; sometimes a very diffuse, nonlocalized pain is present.[3] As such, a careful physical examination is paramount to the evaluation. In particular, evaluation of hindfoot motion and position is critical and must also be compared with the contralateral side.[5] Limited range of motion in the subtalar joint is consistently reported in studies on tarsal coalition, and subtalar coalitions have the greatest limitation in motion across that joint.[3] Specific attention to hindfoot valgus and varus position is also important, as both planovalgus and cavovarus deformity have been reported (**Fig. 1**A).[3,15] Finally, the peroneal tendons should be closely examined, because peroneal spasm, tenderness, or inflammation may be present.[3,5,10,17]

IMAGING

Standard weight-bearing foot and ankle views constitute the initial radiographic evaluation (see **Fig. 1**B, C). The typical 3 views of the foot may show signs that suggest a subtalar coalition. Specifically, beaking at the talonavicular joint, a broad lateral process of the talus, and/or a narrowing of the joint space in the posterior facet may be seen. Abnormal motion of the subtalar joint may lead to these findings and thus make the clinician suspicious of a subtalar coalition.[12,13,18] Additional signs that may be seen on plain radiographs as described by Crim and Kjeldsberg[19] include a loss of the middle facet, a short neck of the talus, and a dysmorphic sustentaculum tali.[3,19] Finally, the "C sign" has classically been described on lateral radiographs as a circular density formed by the outline of the dome of the talus and the inferior aspect of the sustentaculum.[3,20] Normal alignment of the talus and calcaneus is distorted by their bony connection, leading to the appearance of a "C" on the radiograph. However, the sensitivity and specificity of the C sign are lacking.[5,21] In addition to standard films, coronal alignment may be shown with a weight-bearing hindfoot alignment radiograph.[5] A Harris heel view is also helpful when suspicious of subtalar coalition. In a normal patient, the posterior and middle facets are parallel; patients with greater than 25° angulation of the middle facet away from the posterior facet likely have a subtalar coalition.[5,22]

Although radiographs are very useful in diagnosing subtalar coalitions, more sophisticated imaging is often obtained to assess and treat the pathologic abnormality. CT and magnetic resonance imaging (MRI) are very useful to help diagnose a coalition that may be missed on plain radiographs.[3,23,24] CT is especially useful when evaluating bony coalitions, revealing the size and location of the subtalar coalition.[3,5] MRI is

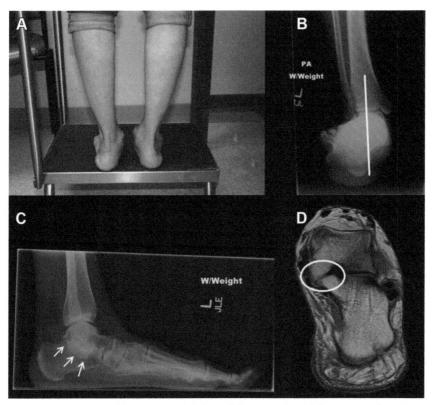

Fig. 1. (*A–D*) A 45-year-old woman with bilateral foot pain (L > R) for greater than 2 years. Pain primarily in the sinus tarsi region. The patient had increasing pain despite conservative treatment for 2 years with CAM walker boot and physical therapy. Her American Orthopaedic Foot and Ankle Society (AOFAS) score was 55. (*A*) Hindfoot view demonstrating bilateral pes planovalgus deformity. (*B*) Weight-bearing left hindfoot alignment view radiograph with plumb line demonstrating hind foot valgus. (*C*) Weight-bearing left lateral radiograph demonstrating "C" sign (*arrows*). (*D*) Axial T1 MRI demonstrating middle facet talocalcaneal coalition (*circle*). (*From* Thorpe SW, Wukich DK. Tarsal coalitions in the adult population: does treatment differ from the adolescent? Foot Ankle Clin 2012;17:195–204; with permission.)

helpful in diagnosing fibrous or cartilaginous coalitions and can also aid the clinician in management by revealing concomitant chondral, ligamentous, or tendon damage (see **Fig. 1**D).[3,5] Furthermore, MRI may show hyperintensity of the bone marrow in the setting of a subtalar coalition.[5,25] Thus, knowledge from CT and MRI may guide the management of the patient.

NONOPERATIVE TREATMENT

Typically, an injury to the union between the talus and calcaneus will cause the subtalar coalition to become symptomatic.[5] A trial of nonoperative treatment is initially indicated. A multimodal approach includes the use of nonsteroidal anti-inflammatory drugs, activity modification, orthoses, such as those from the University of California-Berkeley Laboratories, and physical therapy.[3,5,12] Casting, possibly immobilization in a removable cast boot for 4 to 6 weeks, may also be very effective and is often tried if the above-mentioned measures fail.[12] As Leonard[7] suggested in

1974, most coalitions become symptomatic because of a recent trauma; therefore, nonoperative treatment may be very effective in alleviating the pain.[3,7,12] Results of nonoperative treatment in adults have, however, been variable. Although Varner and Michelson[12] showed 67% efficacy in treating adult tarsal coalitions conservatively, Cohen and colleagues[26] only had success treating 3 of 19 patients nonoperatively.[26] Furthermore, there is a paucity of data on conservative treatment of tarsal coalitions in adults, and no study is isolated to the subtalar coalition. In addition, it is not known what the natural history is of the asymptomatic subtalar coalition.[5] Therefore, it is difficult to draw any firm conclusions.

OPERATIVE TREATMENT

If a patient remains symptomatic despite a trial of conservative treatment, operative intervention is indicated. The 2 main surgical options include resection of the coalition and surgical fusion.[3] There is considerable debate in the literature as to which is the more appropriate choice. Age, size of the coalition, alignment of the hindfoot, assessment of range of motion of the affected joint, bone versus cartilaginous coalition, and presence of arthritic changes in the subtalar and adjacent joints are all important considerations. In addition, after choosing which option to pursue, the surgeon must make further decisions, including interposition into the resection bed and method of fusion in the arthrodesis site. The use of Amniox Clarix has been used as an interposition recently with success. Although the studies are not completed, interim data suggest this as a viable option. After coalition resection, the Clarix is applied, which promotes healing without scar formation (**Figs. 2** and **3**).

As previously discussed, after deciding on surgical intervention, the surgeon should obtain a CT scan to evaluate both the size of the coalition and the presence of arthritis in the subtalar and adjacent joints.[5,27] If arthritic change is present, fusion is the treatment of choice.[3,5] It should be noted that the presence of talar beaking has been theorized to be a dorsal traction spur from the talonavicular ligament and not indicative of concomitant arthrosis.[28] Several studies have reported good to excellent results despite the presence of talar beaking after resection of the coalition.[29–31]

With regard to size of the coalition, several studies have suggested that subtalar coalitions that involve greater than 50% of the posterior facet should be fused. Although Scranton[32] initially chose this percentage seemingly arbitrarily,[3,32] it has been further

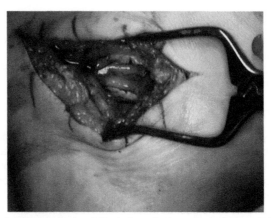

Fig. 2. Intraoperative photograph of Clarix (Amniox) applied after coalition resection.

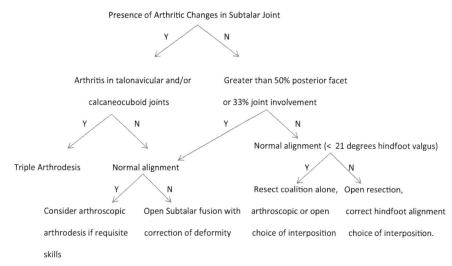

Presence of Arthritic Changes in Subtalar Joint

Y / N

Arthritis in talonavicular and/or calcaneocuboid joints   Greater than 50% posterior facet or 33% joint involvement

Y / N   Y / N

Normal alignment (< 21 degrees hindfoot valgus)

Triple Arthrodesis   Normal alignment

Y / N   Y / N

Consider arthroscopic   Open Subtalar fusion with   Resect coalition alone,   Open resection,

arthrodesis if requisite   correction of deformity   arthroscopic or open   correct hindfoot alignment

skills   choice of interposition   choice of interposition.

Fig. 3. Algorithm for the surgical management of adult subtalar coalition.

supported by the research of Wilde and colleagues,[29] who reported poorer outcomes when resection was perform in patients whose coalition involved greater than 50% of the posterior facet. The research of Luhmann and Schonecker[27] in the pediatric population also demonstrated similar results, although they recommended excision despite the size of the coalition. In addition to posterior facet involvement, the surgeon must carefully look at the entire subtalar joint. If greater than 33% of the joint is affected by the coalition, patients tend to have poor results if resection is chosen.[33] In the series of Philbin and colleagues[34] of 7 patients who had resection of a coalition of the middle facet, one patient had a coalition greater than 50% of the joint, and this patient did not improve. The only factor in their series that appeared to significantly impact outcome, however, was the cartilaginous content of the coalition, because those with a greater degree of normal cartilage tended to have better outcomes.[34]

Hindfoot alignment has also been shown to affect results of surgical intervention. In particular, severe hindfoot valgus portends unsatisfactory outcomes. Wilde and colleagues[29] demonstrated poor results when hindfoot alignment was greater than 16° valgus, while Luhmann and Schonecker[27] found that patients with 21° hindfoot valgus did worse. As such, several case series have looked at concurrent correction of the hindfoot along with resection of the coalition. Luhmann and Schonecker[27] suggested that either a medial displacing calcaneal osteotomy or a lateral column lengthening be used after resection to more appropriately align the hindfoot. If there was good subtalar motion following resection, they lengthened the lateral column; if it was restricted, they performed a medial displacement calcaneal osteotomy.[27] Lisella and colleagues[35] recently reported on 7 patients who had excellent correction of the arch with a hindfoot reconstruction in addition to resection of the coalition.[35] Furthermore, Mosca and Bevan[36] suggested in the pediatric population that deformity correction is as important as the resection of the coalition. Their series of patients who underwent both a lateral column lengthening through the calcaneus and an Achilles lengthening had excellent results with pain relief and deformity correction.[36] Others have reported the use of a subtalar arthroereisis to restore the alignment of the calcaneus and talus following resection.[37] Although the data are limited to a small number of level IV studies, patients who have significant hindfoot valgus appear to do less well, and severe deformities should be addressed simultaneously. However, with the available literature, the best method to correct residual hindfoot alignment is not clear and should be tailored to both the patient and the specific deformity.[3] A recent long-term follow-up of pediatric patients who underwent resection suggested that neither size greater or less than 50% and alignment greater or less than 16° matters; however, this may not necessarily be applicable to the adult population.[38]

The additional question that arises following resection of a subtalar coalition is whether to interpose tissue or graft in its place. Although some surgeons have obtained good results without placing any material in the resected space,[30] many others have interposed tissue. Fat grafts have been harvested locally from behind the calcaneus with good results.[32,39] This local fat graft may even be pedicled and sutured in place.[40] Fat may also be taken from the buttocks or abdomen.[41] In adolescents, a portion of the flexor hallucis longus tendon has also been interposed, with the patients again doing very well.[42,43] Bone wax in pediatric patients[44] and fibrin glue in both adolescents and young adults[45] have also been introduced with good to excellent results. Based on level IV studies, Lemley and colleagues[3] recommended that some type of interposed tissue should be placed in the subtalar space following resection.[3] At the current time, the ideal interposition graft is not known.

As arthroscopic techniques have advanced, surgeons have introduced arthroscopy in the treatment of subtalar coalitions, in both arthrodesis and resection. Bonasia and colleagues[46] were concerned with the limitations of open resection and introduced a technique to resect a subtalar coalition using subtalar arthroscopy from a posterior approach with the patient prone. Specifically, they thought that subtalar arthroscopy provided excellent visualization of the entire subtalar joint, especially the posterior facet, which may not be well visualized with an open approach. Furthermore, arthroscopy allowed the surgeon to assess the extent of the resection and the presence of arthritis. They do acknowledge, however, the steep learning curve and difficulty using interposition material. They recommend consideration of arthroscopic excision if the coalition is located in the posterior facet, if there are adequate posterior tibial pulses, and if there have been no prior hindfoot surgeries.[46] Posterior arthroscopy has also been used for arthrodesis in patients with a subtalar coalition and relatively normal alignment. However, 2 patients in a recent series had lateral malleolar impingement postoperatively.[47] In addition, there were difficulties with distraction of the subtalar joint. As such, the authors recommended a 3-portal technique as described by Beimers and colleagues.[47] In the 3-portal technique, an accessory portal is placed across the sinus tarsi to aid in opening the joint space and in debriding the cartilage in the anterior part of the posterior facet.[48] Surgeons with extensive arthroscopic experience may thus choose to treat adults with subtalar coalitions arthroscopically for either fusion or resection of the coalition.

When arthrodesis is chosen, the surgeon must carefully assess the subtalar joint as well as the rest of the hindfoot. If the arthritis is isolated to the subtalar joint, isolated fusion is generally accepted. CT and/or MRI studies before surgery are recommended; however, if there is more extensive articular damage, triple arthrodesis of the subtalar, talonavicular, and calcaneocuboid joints is performed.[3,5,12,28,32] In addition, triple arthrodesis has been used consistently in salvage situations. Patients with significant preoperative hindfoot valgus must also be carefully evaluated because fusion of the subtalar joint in slight valgus may result in a forefoot varus position, which must be corrected with a triple arthrodesis to obtain a plantigrade foot. In the presence of persistent pain after excision, recurrent bone formation, or deterioration of the joint, triple arthrodesis has generally been accepted.[3,27]

SUMMARY

In summary, there remains a dearth of primary research on subtalar coalitions in the adult population. Drawing from a mix of adult and adolescent studies, however, adults with a subtalar coalition can be confidently managed. Because the coalition in an adult is often discovered incidentally after injury, or may have been asymptomatic for a long period of time, initial conservative management may be successful.[5] When a patient fails nonoperative treatment, an algorithm for operative treatment is proposed. In the presence of arthritic change, arthrodesis should be offered to the patient. It may be done arthroscopically if isolated to the subtalar joint, if alignment is appropriate, and if the surgeon has the requisite technical skills. If arthritis is present in talonavicular and/or calcaneocuboid joints, these should be included in the fusion. If no arthritis is present, but the coalition involves more than 50% of the posterior facet or more than 33% of the entire subtalar joint, fusion should also strongly be considered. If the coalition is smaller, however, resection may be attempted, either open or arthroscopically. Local tissue graft or commercial product such as fibrin glue or bone wax may be interposed. Severe malalignment of the hindfoot, particularly significant hindfoot valgus, should be corrected concurrently or the outcomes tend to be worse. However, patients undergoing a resection should be cautioned that outcomes may not be predictable, and they may ultimately need a fusion procedure in the future.

REFERENCES

1. Stormont DM, Peterson HA. The relative incidence of tarsal coalition. Clin Orthop Relat Res 1983;(181):28–36.
2. Kulik SA Jr, Clanton TO. Tarsal coalition. Foot Ankle Int 1996;17(5):286–96.
3. Lemley F, Berlet G, Hill K, et al. Current concepts review: tarsal coalition. Foot Ankle Int 2006;27(12):1163–9.
4. Zaw H, Calder JD. Tarsal coalitions. Foot Ankle Clin N Am 2010;15:349–64.
5. Thorpe SW, Wukich DK. Tarsal coalitions in the adult population: does treatment differ from the adolescent. Foot Ankle Clin N Am 2012;17:195–204.
6. Solomon LB, Ruhli FJ, Taylor J, et al. A dissection and computer tomography study of tarsal coalitions in 100 cadaveric feet. J Orthop Res 2003;21:352–8.
7. Leonard MA. The inheritance of tarsal coalition and its relationship to spastic flat foot. J Bone Joint Surg Br 1974;56:520–6.
8. Harris BJ. Anomalous structures in the developing human foot. Anat Rec 1955; 121:399.
9. Leboucq H. De la soudyre congenitale de certains os du tarse. Bull Acad R Med Belg 1890;4:103–12 [in French].
10. Mosier KM, Asher M. Tarsal coalitions and peroneal spastic flatfoot: a review. J Bone Joint Surg Am 1984;66:976–84.
11. Harris RI, Beath T. Etiology of peroneal spastic flat foot. J Bone Joint Surg Br 1948;20:624–34.
12. Varner KE, Michelson JD. Tarsal coalition in adults. Foot Ankle Int 2000;21: 669–72.
13. Rankin EA, Baker GI. Rigid flatfoot in the young adult. Clin Orthop Relat Res 1974;(104):244–8.
14. Hughes A, Brown R. Talar body fracture associated with unrecognized talocalcaneal coalition. Foot Ankle Surg 2010;16(2):e4–7.
15. Stuecker RD, Bennett JT. Tarsal coalition presenting as a pes cavo-varus deformity: report of three cases and review of the literature. Foot Ankle Int 1993;14: 540–4.

16. Wahnert D, Gruneweller N, Evers J, et al. An unusual cause of ankle pain: fracture of a talocalcaneal coalition as a differential diagnosis in an acute ankle sprain: a case report and literature review. BMC Musculoskelet Disord 2013;14:111.

17. Cowell HR. Talocalcaneal coalition and new causes of peroneal spastic flatfoot. Clin Orthop Relat Res 1972;85:16–22.

18. Conway JJ, Cowell HR. Tarsal coalition: clinical significance and roentgenographic demonstration. Radiology 1969;92:799.

19. Crim J, Kjeldsberg K. Radiographic diagnosis of tarsal coalition. AJR Am J Roentgenol 2004;18:323–8.

20. Lateur LM, Van Hoe LR, Van Ghillewe KV, et al. Subtalar coalition: diagnosis with the C sign on lateral radiographs of the ankle. Radiology 1994;193:847–51.

21. Brown RR, Rosenberg ZS, Thonhill BA. The C sign: more specific for flatfoot deformity than subtalar coalition. Skeletal Radiol 2001;30:84–7.

22. Cowell HR, Elener V. Rigid painful flatfoot secondary to tarsal coalition. Clin Orthop Relat Res 1983;(177):54–60.

23. Herzenberg JE, Goldner JL, Martinez S, et al. Computerized tomography of talocalcaneal tarsal coalition: a clinical and anatomic study. Foot Ankle Int 1986;6:273–88.

24. Pineda C, Resnick D, Greenway G. Diagnosis of tarsal coalition with computed tomography. Clin Orthop Relat Res 1986;(208):282–8.

25. Sijbrandi ES, van Gils AP, de Lange EE, et al. Bone marrow ill-defined hyperintensities with tarsal coalition: MR imaging findings. Eur J Radiol 2002;43:61–5.

26. Cohen BE, Davis WH, Anderson RB. Success of calcaneonavicular coalition resection in the adult population. Foot Ankle Int 1996;15:569–72.

27. Luhmann SJ, Schonecker PL. Symptomatic talocalcaneal resection: indications and results. J Pediatr Orthop 1998;18:748–54.

28. Swiontkowski MF, Scranton PE, Hansen S. Tarsal coalitions: long-term results of surgical treatment. J Pediatr Orthop 1983;3:287–92.

29. Wilde PH, Torode IP, Dickens DR, et al. Resection for symptomatic talocalcaneal coalition. J Bone Joint Surg Br 1994;76:797–801.

30. Kitaoka HB, Wikenheiser MA, Shaughnessy WJ, et al. Gait abnormalities following resection of talocalcaneal coalition. J Bone Joint Surg Am 1997;79:369–74.

31. McCormack TJ, Olney B, Asher M. Talocalcaneal coalition resection: a 10-year follow-up. J Pediatr Orthopp 1997;17:13–5.

32. Scranton PE. Treatment of symptomatic talocalcaneal coalition. J Bone Joint Surg Am 1987;69:533–9.

33. Comfort TK, Johnson LO. Resection for symptomatic talocalcaneal coalition. J Pediatr Orthopp 1998;18:283–8.

34. Philbin TM, Homan B, Hill K, et al. Results of resection for middle facet tarsal coalitions in adults. Foot Ankle Spec 2008;1:344–9.

35. Lisella JM, Bellapianta JM, Manoli A. Tarsal coalition resection with pes planovalgus hindfoot reconstruction. J Surg Orthop Adv 2011;20(2):102–5.

36. Mosca VS, Bevan WP. Talocalcaneal tarsal coalitions and the calcaneal lengthening osteotomy: the role of deformity correction. J Bone Joint Surg Am 2012;94:1584–94.

37. Giannini S, Ceccarelli F, Vannini F, et al. Operative treatment of flatfoot with talocalcaneal coalition. Clin Orthop Relat Res 2003;(411):178–87.

38. Khosbin A, Law PL, Caspi L, et al. Long term functional outcomes of resected tarsal coalitions. Foot Ankle Int 2013;34:1370–5.

39. Salomao O, Napli MM, de Carvalho AE, et al. Talocalcaneal coalition: diagnosis and surgical management. Foot Ankle Int 1992;13:251–6.

40. Imajima Y, Takao M, Miyamoto W, et al. Midterm outcome of talocalcaneal coalition treated with interposition of a pedicle fatty flap after resection. Foot Ankle Int 2012;33:226–30.
41. Gantsoudes GD, Roocroft JH, Mubarak SJ. Treatment of talocalcaneal coalitions. J Pediatr Orthop 2012;31(3):301–7.
42. Kumar MD, Guille JT, Lee MS, et al. Osseous and nonosseous coalition of the mddle facet of the talocalcaneal joint. J Bone Joint Surg Am 1992;74:529–35.
43. Raikin S, Cooperman DR, Thompson GH. Interposition of the split flexor hallucis longus tendon after resection of a coalition of the middle facet of the talocalcaneal joint. J Bone Joint Surg Am 1999;81:11–9.
44. Westberry DE, Davids JR, Oros W. Surgical management of symptomatic talocalcaneal coalitions by resection of the sustentaculum tali. J Pediatr Orthop 2003;23:493–7.
45. Weatherall JM, Price AE. Fibrin glue as interposition graft for tarsal coalition. Am J Orthop 2013;42(1):26–9.
46. Bonasia DE, Phisitkul P, Saltzman CL, et al. Athroscopic resection of talocalcaneal coalitions. Arthroscopy 2011;27(3):430–5.
47. Albert A, Deleu PA, Leemrijse T, et al. Posterior arthroscopic arthrodesis: ten cases at one-year follow-up. Orthop Traumatol Surg Res 2011;97:401–5.
48. Beimers L, De Leeuw PA, Van Dijk CN. A 3-portal approach for arthroscopic subtalar arthrodesis. Knee Surg Sports Traumatol Arthrosc 2009;17:830–4.

The Spectrum of Indications for Subtalar Joint Arthrodesis

Ettore Vulcano, MD[a],*, J. Kent Ellington, MD, MS[b],
Mark S. Myerson, MD[c]

KEYWORDS

- Subtalar joint fusion • Sinus tarsi incision • Medial extensile
- Lateral approach incision • Subtalar fusion • Bone block fusion • Subtalar nonunion

KEY POINTS

- Subtalar fusion can be performed in isolation or in association with other procedures, and it may be done in situ or with a bone block to restore optimal foot and ankle alignment.
- The subtalar joint can be difficult to identify and open, and use of fluoroscopy to correctly locate the joint and laminar spreaders to gradually pry the space open is recommended.
- Symptoms at the subtalar joint may not necessarily be related to intrinsic problems of the joint.

INTRODUCTION

The indications for subtalar fusion are numerous, ranging from congenital to acquired deformities. The most commonly encountered subtalar pathologies include posttraumatic arthritis,[1,2] comminuted calcaneal fractures,[3] primary arthritis,[4] talocalcaneal coalitions,[4,5] and posterior tibial tendon dysfunction.[6,7]

   The preferred surgical approaches are the sinus tarsi incision, the medial incision, and the extensile lateral approach. The choice of one over the other depends on the underlying pathology, previous surgeries, associated foot pathologies, soft tissue quality, and medical comorbidities. Ideally, the sinus tarsi approach should always be preferred to limit the risk of wound dehiscence, especially if previous surgeries were performed (ie, open reduction and internal fixation [ORIF] of a calcaneus fracture). Nonetheless, complex deformities such as a severe hindfoot valgus may benefit from a medial approach to avoid wound closure complications on the lateral aspect of

The authors have nothing to disclose.
[a] The Institute for Foot and Ankle Reconstruction, Mercy Medical Center, 301 Saint Paul Street, Baltimore, MD 21202, USA; [b] OrthoCarolina, Foot and Ankle Institute, 2001 Vail Avenue, Charlotte, NC 28207, USA; [c] The Institute for Foot and Ankle Reconstruction, Mercy Medical Center, Baltimore, MD, USA
* Corresponding author.
E-mail address: ettorevulcano@hotmail.com

Foot Ankle Clin N Am 20 (2015) 293–310
http://dx.doi.org/10.1016/j.fcl.2015.02.002
1083-7515/15/$ – see front matter © 2015 Elsevier Inc. All rights reserved.

the hindfoot. Conversely, patients who present with subtalar arthritis, subfibular impingement secondary to calcaneus widening, and peroneal tendon pathology, may have to be treated through a lateral extensile incision to decompress subfibular impingement.

There are 2 types of subtalar fusion procedures: fusion performed in situ and a bone block arthrodesis with structural grafting to restore the height of the hindfoot. Subtalar fusion may be performed alone or in conjunction with other procedures to address coexisting deformities or pathologies that are often encountered in patients with subtalar arthritis: peroneal or flexor hallucis longus tendinopathies, tarsal tunnel syndrome, ankle instability, or malalignment requiring the addition of a calcaneal osteotomy.

Finally, the planning of a subtalar fusion requires a thorough assessment of any risk factors for nonunion. These may include revision surgery, talus avascular necrosis, posttraumatic arthritis, smoking, rheumatoid arthritis, systemic lupus erythematosus or other autoimmune disorders, and diabetes.[8–10] Routine use of biologic or structural augments to facilitate bone healing is not necessary if a meticulous joint preparation and rigid fixation with compression are used. However, high-risk patients may benefit from bone grafting, bone morphogenetic proteins, demineralized bone matrix, or mesenchymal stem cells to prevent such a cumbersome complication.

This report discusses 6 clinical conditions that required a subtalar fusion. The indications, surgical approach, and associated procedures are discussed.

Case 1—Subtalar Joint Middle Facet Coalition

A healthy 26-year-old woman presented with bilateral foot pain after prolonged weight bearing and sporting activities. The pain was localized at the lateral aspect of the hindfoot and sinus tarsi.

On physical examination she presented with bilateral pes planovalgus and rigid hindfoot valgus. Weight bearing radiographs of both feet and ankles confirmed bilateral middle facet coalitions and a significant talar neck osteophyte (**Fig. 1**). Despite our reluctance, the patient requested having both feet treated at the same time. The surgical plan consisted of an in situ subtalar fusion, a cotton osteotomy of the first metatarsal, and exostectomy of the talar neck osteophyte.

The patient was positioned prone on the operating table in a "frog leg" position (**Fig. 2**). A sinus tarsi incision was made to access the subtalar joint. We prefer to avoid an aggressive sinus tarsi debridement to prevent devascularization; however, middle facet coalitions are particularly tedious to treat, as they make the exposure of the posterior facet difficult. At times, the subtalar joint may be obliterated to the point that one can mistakenly fall into the ankle joint instead. Placing a small retractor over the peroneal tendons and behind the tuberosity will make the posterior facet more visible and accessible for debridement. We also insert an osteotome into the subtalar space and confirm the position fluoroscopically. Then the middle facet coalition is taken down with the osteotome and a mallet. As the coalition is gradually and carefully removed, avoiding damage to the medial neurovascular and tendon structures, a laminar spreader inserted into the sinus tarsi is gradually opened (**Fig. 3**). Once the subtalar joint has been fully exposed and prepared, it can be provisionally fixed with guide pins inserted perpendicularly to the joint from anterior to posterior and from posterior to anterior. The choice of inserting at least 1 of the 2 7.0-mm screws from anterior to posterior is to decrease the odds of the patient having heel pain postoperatively, which may occur even with headless screws. Before fixation, the calcaneus should be internally rotated slightly under the talus to correct the hindfoot valgus. After the subtalar joint was fused, a second longitudinal incision was made over the talar

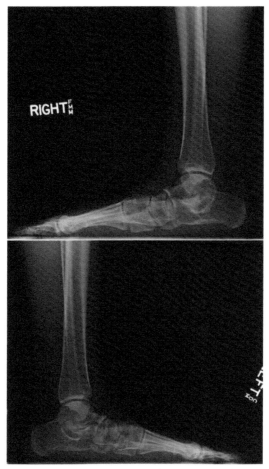

Fig. 1. Preoperative weight bearing radiographs show bilateral flatfoot deformity, middle facet coalition, and talar neck beaking.

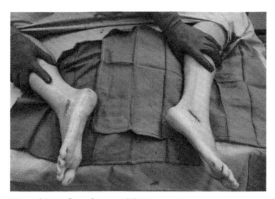

Fig. 2. Patient positioned in a frog-leg position.

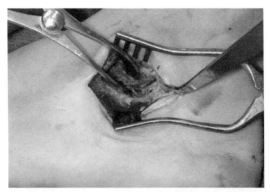

Fig. 3. A small retractor over the peroneal tendons and behind the tuberosity make the posterior facet more visible and accessible for debridement. A laminar spreader inserted into the sinus tarsi greatly facilitates the exposure and preparation of the joint.

neck extending to the first tarsometatarsal joint. The talar neck osteophyte was removed, and the medial column was plantarflexed through a medial cuneiform opening wedge osteotomy (**Fig. 4**).

Case 2—Subtalar Joint Arthritis with Anterior Ankle Impingement

This is a case of a 57-year-old gentleman with right ankle and hindfoot pain for many years. His surgical history was significant for bilateral total knee replacements for genu varum. On examination, the patient had a neutral knee alignment with mild distal tibia vara. There was inversion through the subtalar joint bilaterally with no motion on the right. The ankle joint had 5° of dorsiflexion and about 30° of plantar flexion. Weight bearing radiographs of the ankles showed severe right subtalar arthritis with flattening of the talar declination angle leading to ankle arthritis with significant anterior impingement (**Fig. 5**).

The operative plan for this patient consisted of a bone block arthrodesis of the subtalar joint to restore pitch and subtalar space and an anterior ankle cheilectomy. We

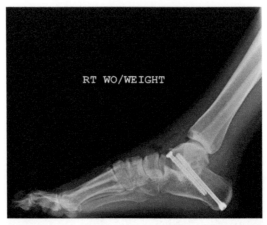

RT WO/WEIGHT

Fig. 4. Postoperative simulated weight bearing radiograph shows correction of the alignment of the foot.

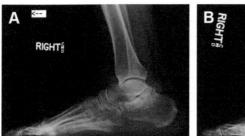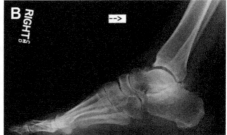

Fig. 5. Flexion (*A*) and extension (*B*) lateral views of the right ankle. Note the loss of talar declination and the anterior ankle impingement.

also opted to add autologous bone marrow aspirate concentrate to improve integration of the bone block allograft.

The patient was positioned on the left lateral decubitus. A longitudinal incision was made just lateral to the tendo Achilles along the posterolateral aspect of the ankle joint down to the heel. The incision for a bone block must be vertical. If any incision is placed in the longitudinal plane of the foot and an increase in the height of the hindfoot is created, a wound dehiscence will likely occur.

Once the ankle and subtalar joints were identified both under direct visualization and fluoroscopy, a curved osteotomy was inserted into the posterior facet. Laminar spreaders were used to gradually open the joint and to increase the talar declination angle (**Fig. 6**). As the posterior facet is prepared, it should be kept in mind that the middle facet must also be exposed and denuded of cartilage to adequately accept the bone graft. Once the desired talar declination angle was restored, the bone graft was inserted and the laminar spreader removed.

Fixation was achieved with 2 cannulated 7.0-mm screws inserted from anterior to posterior and from posterior to anterior, respectively. Once the subtalar bone block fusion was completed, an anterolateral ankle mini arthrotomy was used to perform the anterior ankle cheilectomy.

Although malunion is rare with in situ fusion, it is a common complication of bone block arthrodesis. The heel should be well aligned under the leg, and the forefoot must be plantigrade. Having the patient in the lateral decubitus is unfortunately not helpful to assess the correct alignment of the hindfoot-forefoot-knee. If in doubt, it is better to have the heel in slight valgus. Another problem with distraction of the

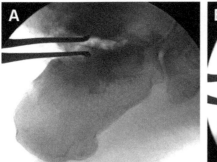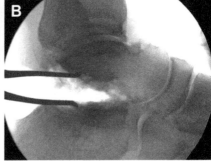

Fig. 6. (*A*) fluoroscopic intraoperative image shows initial subtalar joint exposure and opening. (*B*) Progressive opening of the subtalar joint to restore a normal talar declination angle.

subtalar joint is that the laminar spreader tends to align the calcaneus into varus. To prevent this, the bone graft can be modeled to be higher on the medial side than on the lateral side. This action may not be necessary if addressing a flatfoot deformity in which correction of the hindfoot valgus is desirable.

Case 3—Subtalar Coalition with Loss of Talar Height

A 54-year-old male martial arts instructor presented with a longstanding history of bilateral foot pain worse on the right side. He had about 25° of ankle range of motion and no subtalar joint motion. The most significant pain was located at the subtalar joint and in the subfibular region. Weight bearing ankle radiographs and a weight bearing computed tomography (CT) scan showed severe arthritis of the subtalar joint and bilateral talocalcaneal coalitions (**Figs. 7** and **8**). There was also decreased height of the talus with a flat talar declination angle and subfibular impingement. Hindfoot alignment showed 20° of valgus on the right side. Our operative plan consisted of a bone block fusion of the subtalar joint with the addition of autologous bone marrow aspirate concentrate, percutaneous Achilles tendon lengthening, and anterior ankle cheilectomy.

The patient was positioned on his left side, and a longitudinal skin incision was made for a posterolateral approach to the ankle. Care should be taken so as not to injure the sural nerve. As with all cases of subfibular impingement, the peroneal tendon sheath must be opened and the tendons examined for tears. The subtalar joint is often difficult to localize. We recommend fluoroscopic examination in any case.

Once the subtalar joint was identified, prying of the joint with an osteotome first, followed by a laminar spreader, helped with exposing the joint. The calcaneus was then reduced under the talus, which, in turn, had its declination angle restored to normal, and the bone wedge—enriched with bone marrow aspirate—was inserted into the joint. At this point, the tension in the Achilles tendon was noted to create not only some difficulty with the reduction maneuvers but was also limiting ankle dorsiflexion. As planned preoperatively, a percutaneous lengthening of the tendo Achilles was

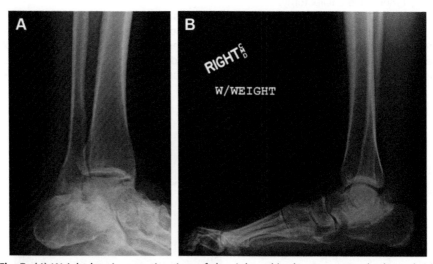

Fig. 7. (A) Weight bearing mortise view of the right ankle shows severe subtalar arthritis and subfibular impingement. (B) Weight bearing lateral view of the ankle shows the anterior ankle impingement and the loss of talar height with flattening.

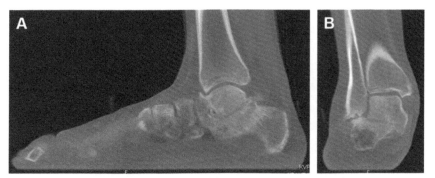

Fig. 8. (A) Weight bearing CT scan sagittal view shows severe subtalar arthritis and talocalcaneal coalition and anterior ankle impingement. (B) Weight bearing CT coronal view of the ankle shows the significant subfibular impingement.

performed. Our aim was to achieve about 10° of ankle dorsiflexion with the bone block in place. Fixation of the bone block fusion was obtained with two 7.0-mm cannulated screws. Following these procedures, an anteromedial mini arthrotomy was used to perform a tibial and talar neck cheilectomy to address the ankle impingement (**Fig. 9**).

Case 4—Posttraumatic Subtalar Arthritis with Severe Subfibular Impingement and Peroneal Dislocation

A 58-year-old man presented to our clinic with severe foot pain that had progressively worsened over the years. He had undergone ORIF for a calcaneus fracture 30 years prior after falling from a tree. On examination he had good lower limb alignment but obvious widening of his left heel. His peroneal tendons were dislocated, and there were signs of subfibular impingement. There was a lateral surgical scar and numbness in the sural nerve distribution. His ankle joint moved well, but the subtalar (ST) joint was rigid.

Weight bearing ankle radiographs and weight bearing CT scan (**Figs. 10** and **11**) confirmed severe subtalar joint arthritis but reasonable alignment of the hindfoot. The studies also found significant subfibular impingement.

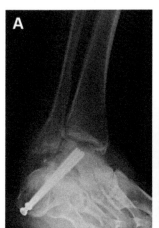
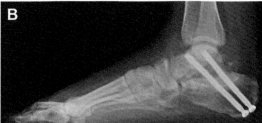

Fig. 9. (A) Postoperative weight bearing mortise view of the right ankle shows fusion of the bone block arthrodesis and resolution of the subfibular impingement. (B) Postoperative weight bearing lateral view of the ankle shows correction of the talar declination angle.

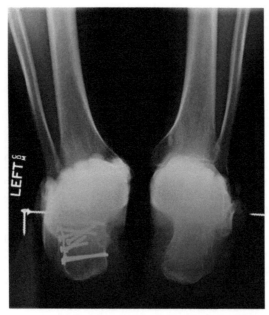

Fig. 10. Preoperative hindfoot alignment view shows widening of the os calcis.

The surgical plan included removal of the hardware from the calcaneus, calcaneal exostectomy, and subtalar fusion. Because a previous surgery had been performed, we also opted to add bone morphogenetic protein 2 to facilitate bone healing (**Fig. 12**).

The patient was positioned in a lateral decubitus. The previous L-shaped extensile incision was used to approach the calcaneus and subtalar joint. To preserve the integrity of the flap, it is crucial to handle the latter as one thick soft tissue flap dissecting straight onto bone. After exposure of the calcaneus' lateral surface, there was extensive and massive bony overgrowth with impingement of the calcaneal osteophytes onto the fibula. Using a sharp chisel, the lateral wall of the calcaneus was osteotomized, leading to exposure of the plate, which was then removed. Then, the subtalar joint was identified and opened and prepared for fusion. After preparation of the joint,

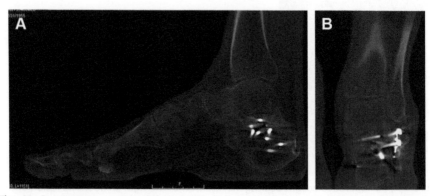

Fig. 11. Preoperative weight bearing CT scan. (*A*) Sagittal view shows severe subtalar arthritis. (*B*) Coronal view shows widening of the calcaneus and subfibular impingement.

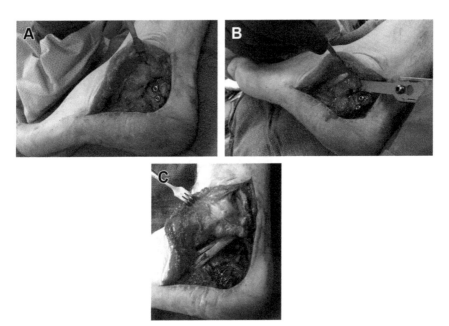

Fig. 12. (*A, B*) Intraoperative photographs shows the massive exostosis over the calcaneus causing subfibular impingement. A sharp chisel was used to clear the lateral wall of the os calcis. Also, note the dislocated peroneal tendons. (*C*) End result with no subfibular impingement and peroneal tendons in place.

our attention turned to the peroneal tendons, which were dislocated anteriorly over the distal fibula. A soft tissue release was done, and they were reduced to their anatomic position. A 2-inch soft tissue fascial flap was raised from the usual peroneal retinaculum, and this was used to keep them in place.

The subtalar joint was fixed with two 7.0-mm screws. An aggressive calcaneus lateral wall debridement was then performed to prevent subfibular impingement. At the completion of the procedure and when bone graft has been packed into the sinus tarsi, care must be taken to ensure that the graft does not exit and fall between the peroneal tendons and the fibula.

Case 5—Calcaneus Fracture Malunion with Talar Subsidence

This is the case of a healthy 52-year-old man with a history of ORIF of a calcaneus fracture. He presented to the clinic with severe foot and ankle pain. On physical examination he had severe valgus deformity of the hindfoot with obvious signs of subfibular impingement. There was no motion at the subtalar joint, and few degrees of ankle range of motion. Weight bearing radiographs of the ankle showed a malunion of the calcaneal fracture with collapse of the talus into the os calcis and a negative talus declination angle (**Fig. 13**). A weight bearing CT scan is useful to plan the correction, particularly if an osteotomy of the calcaneus needs to be performed in conjunction with the realignment subtalar arthrodesis. Given the severity of the deformity we decided to stage surgery: first, removing the hardware, then to correct the severe deformity, we offered the patient a calcaneal osteotomy, subtalar fusion with a massive bone block, and the addition of bone marrow aspirate concentrate. As an alternative to staging the procedures, the hardware can be removed percutaneously and then the posterior incision used to perform the bone block fusion.

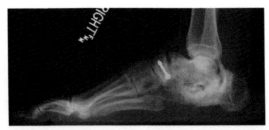

Fig. 13. Weight bearing lateral view radiograph of the ankle shows collapse of the talus into the calcaneus with a negative talar declination angle.

Surgery was performed with the patient on his left side. A longitudinal incision for posterolateral access to the ankle was performed. As with other cases of subtalar bone block, arthrodesis it is paramount to keep the incision straight without curving it in an L-shaped fashion to prevent wound complications. Again, fluoroscopic imaging was crucial to distinguish the ankle from the subtalar joint. After removal of the overhanging bone under the fibula, a guide pin was inserted under fluoroscopy in the plane of the original fracture. This usually is from dorsolateral to plantar and medial at approximately an angle of 30°.

The osteotomy was then performed with an osteotome. Once the osteotomy was complete, the tuberosity was displaced distally and in valgus. Often, loosening of the surrounding soft tissues is required to mobilize the posterior tuberosity. This can be achieved by opening the osteotomy with a laminar spreader. However, this will tend to push the posterior tuberosity into varus. Before stabilizing the osteotomy with guide pins, the correct alignment of the hindfoot must be checked to avoid valgus-varus malalignment.

A curved osteotome followed by laminar spreaders were used to open the subtalar space gradually until a normal declination angle of the talus was restored. Once the desired correction was achieved, a massive bone block enriched with autologous bone marrow aspirate was inserted in the subtalar space. At this point, particular attention must be made not to lose the reduction of the calcaneal osteotomy. Multiple guide pins in the tuberosity extending up into various parts of the calcaneus and the more anterior portion of the talar neck and head will prevent this.

Ultimately, the osteotomy and bone block fusion were stabilized with a fully threaded cannulated 7.0-mm screw (**Fig. 14**).

Case 6—Subtalar Instability After Ankle Fusion. Is a Subtalar Fusion Avoidable?

A 50-year-old woman who had undergone an ankle fusion 6 years prior presented with midfoot pain and difficulty walking on uneven terrains. On physical examination she had a neutral foot-ankle alignment. Range of motion of the subtalar joint was only

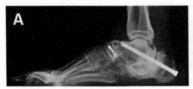
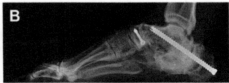

Fig. 14. Postoperative weight bearing (A) flexion and (B) extension lateral views of the ankle. Note the correction of the foot and ankle alignment and the restoration of ankle range of motion.

mildly decreased. Weight bearing ankle radiographs were not impressive other than some initial signs of subtalar arthritis with compression at the posterior facet (**Fig. 15**). However, dorsiflexion and plantarflexion lateral views showed instability at the subtalar joint (**Fig. 16**). The ankle had malunion secondary to fixation of the talus in excessive plantarflexion. The subtalar joint tries to compensate for ankle deformities, as in this patient, but in this case was beginning to show signs of overload. Therefore, we thought we could salvage the subtalar joint by revising the ankle fusion.

A standard anterior approach to the ankle was chosen to perform a closing wedge osteotomy of the distal tibia. First, the hardware from the previous surgery was removed. The osteotomy was planned at the center of rotation of angulation (CORA) of the deformity (**Fig. 17**). The CORA is located at the intersection of 2 lines representing the mechanical axes of the proximal and distal segments of the deformity. A closing wedge osteotomy at the level of the CORA allows for complete realignment of the ankle. If the osteotomy is made proximal or distal to the CORA, the center of the ankle translates relative to the mechanical axis of the tibia and creates an unnecessary shift of loads and a clinically obvious zigzag deformity. When the cuts are made, attention must be made to avoid violation of the posterior cortex that would cause instability of the osteotomy. Finally, we fixed the latter with an anterolateral compression plate (**Fig. 18**). Correct realignment of the ankle resulted in decompression of the subtalar joint and restoration of the midfoot biomechanics, with complete resolution of the patient's symptoms.

Case 7—Subtalar Arthritis and Ankle Fusion Malunion

A healthy 49-year-old man with a previous ankle fusion performed 8 years ago presented to the clinic with severe lateral foot pain. Pain was related to weight bearing and activity. He had been braced in the past with decreasing success in pain control and had a subtalar injection that alleviated his pain for 1 month.

On physical examination, his hindfoot was in valgus while standing, and on seated examination his hindfoot motion was rigid (**Fig. 19**). Radiographs showed an ankle arthrodesis valgus malunion with hindfoot collapse and subtalar arthrosis (**Fig. 20**). Weight bearing CT scan highlighted this and also showed talonavicular involvement (currently fairly asymptomatic) (**Fig. 21**).

Although surgery on this patient is pending, this case highlights the importance of appropriate position during the ankle arthrodesis procedure. This patient went on to rapid subtalar degeneration caused by an ankle malunion.

Case 8—Ankle Fusion and Sinus Tarsi Pain in the Active Patient

Contrary to the previous patient, this patient is a 60-year-old woman that underwent an ankle arthrodesis 25 years ago (**Fig. 22**). She presented to the clinic with sinus tarsi pain that responded well to subtalar injections over several years. She was an avid

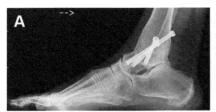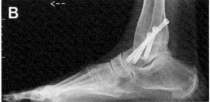

Fig. 15. Preoperative weight bearing (*A*) flexion and (*B*) extension ankle lateral radiographs shows malalignment of the ankle fusion with subtalar instability.

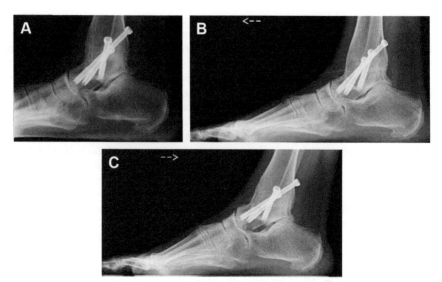

Fig. 16. Preoperative weight bearing lateral ankle view: (*A*) neutral, (*B*) dorsiflexion, (*C*) plantarflexion. Note that the subtalar instability is only observable with dynamic projections. The standard projection only shows mild compression at the subtalar joint.

cyclist and wanted to delay any further surgery. Ultimately, she decided on a subtalar arthrodesis.

The patient was positioned supine with a bump under the ipsilateral hip. A standard sinus tarsi incision was made, and the subtalar joint was debrided. A laminar spreader was placed into the joint to aid in joint visualization and preparation. Once the subtalar joint was fully exposed and prepared, it was provisionally fixed with guide pins inserted perpendicularly to the joint, and it is recommended to obtain purchase in the distal tibia to gain improved fixation (**Fig. 23**). CT scan confirms solid union at 3 months (**Fig. 24**). This case shows that a well-done ankle arthrodesis can preserve

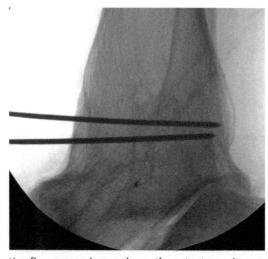

Fig. 17. Intraoperative fluoroscopy image shows the osteotomy sites at the CORA.

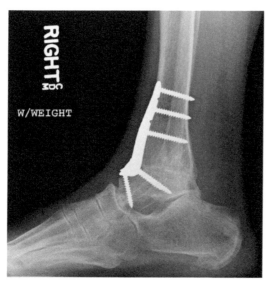

Fig. 18. Postoperative weight bearing radiograph shows correct alignment of the ankle fusion. Clinically, the patient reported complete resolution of the midfoot and hindfoot symptoms.

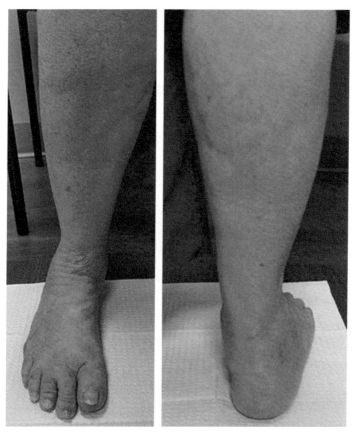

Fig. 19. Preoperative clinical appearance of an ankle valgus malunion with a rigid hindfoot valgus.

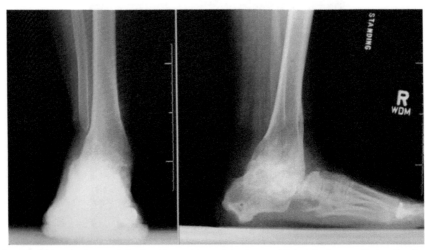

Fig. 20. Preoperative weight bearing anteroposterior and lateral view radiographs show valgus malunion of an ankle fusion and associated hindfoot collapse.

the subtalar joint for a prolonged period. In addition, it should be noted that performing a subtalar arthrodesis below an ankle fusion can lead to a higher nonunion rate owing to the increased lever arm across the subtalar joint. Increased fixation and augmentation with bone graft, coupled with prolonged non–weight bearing and casting, is recommended to reduce the likelihood of a subtalar nonunion. As in this case, bone marrow aspirate mixed with allograft chips were used, and the patient was casted

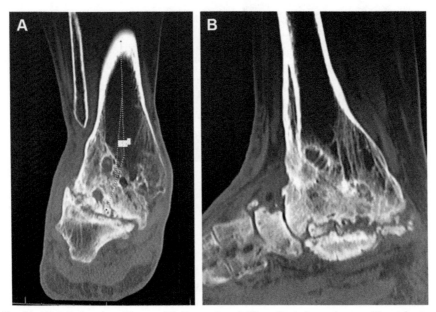

Fig. 21. Weight bearing CT scan. (*A*) Coronal and (*B*) sagittal views show ankle malunion, subtalar arthritis, and talonavicular arthritis.

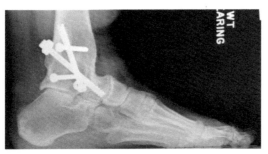

Fig. 22. Preoperative weight bearing lateral view radiograph shows an ankle fusion and subtalar arthritis.

for 8 weeks, then allowed to progressively weight bear after 9 weeks. Luckily, in this case, hardware removal was not necessary.

Case 9—Results of a Minimally Invasive Open Reduction and Internal Fixation for a Calcaneus Fracture

A 45-year-old man sustained a calcaneus fracture 4 years ago and underwent ORIF with a minimally invasive approach (**Fig. 25**). After 3 years he began complaining of si-nus tarsi pain with activity and at work (construction). After short-lived subtalar joint injections and bracing, he elected for subtalar arthrodesis.

The patient was positioned prone. A standard sinus tarsi incision was made, and the subtalar joint was debrided. A laminar spreader was placed into the joint to aid in joint visualization and preparation. The previously placed hardware that is blocking any fix-ation for the subtalar joint was then removed percutaneously. Once the subtalar joint was fully exposed and prepared, it was provisionally fixed with guide pins inserted perpendicularly to the joint (**Fig. 26**).

This case highlights that obtaining proper reduction of a calcaneus fracture leads to an easier subtalar arthrodesis procedure, whereby a distraction bone block is not required nor is residual varus an issue. In addition, it shows that the hardware can be removed percutaneously, and the sinus tarsi approached can still be used, hence, reducing wound healing complications.

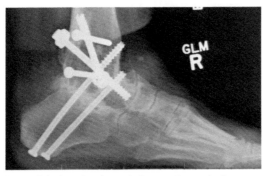

Fig. 23. Postoperative weight bearing lateral view radiograph shows good hindfoot align-ment and fusion across the subtalar joint.

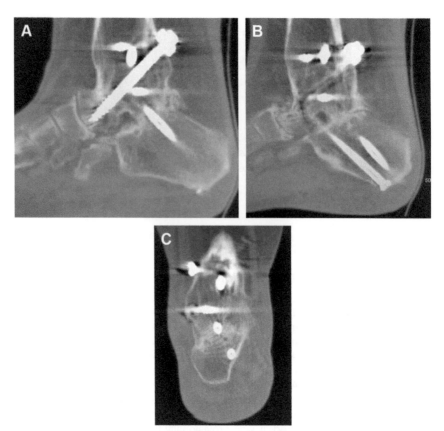

Fig. 24. Postoperative weight bearing CT scan coronal views (*A*, *B*) and sagittal view (*C*) obtained 3 months after surgery. The scans show a solid union across the subtalar joint.

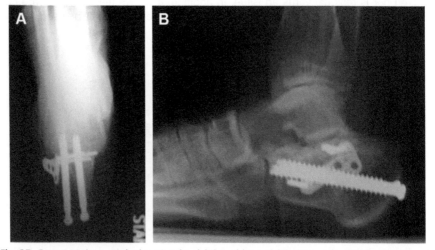

Fig. 25. Preoperative weight bearing heel (*A*) and lateral (*B*) view radiographs show a subtalar arthritis after a previous minimally invasive ORIF of a calcaneus fracture 4 years prior.

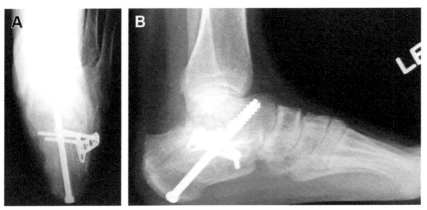

Fig. 26. Postoperative weight bearing heel (*A*) and lateral (*B*) view radiographs show screw orientation and subtalar fusion.

SUMMARY

Subtalar fusion can be performed in isolation or in association with other procedures. It may be done in situ or with a bone block to restore optimal foot and ankle alignment. It is a technically challenging procedure that requires thorough preoperative planning, assessment of patient risk factors, and respect of the soft tissue envelope. The subtalar joint can be difficult to identify and open; therefore, we strongly recommend using fluoroscopy to correctly locate the joint and using laminar spreaders to gradually pry the space open. The hindfoot alignment must be monitored as the subtalar joint is opened, which pushes the calcaneus into varus. This applies particularly to bone block fusions. Unfortunately, it may be difficult to assess when the patient is positioned in a lateral decubitus.

Finally, symptoms at the subtalar joint may not necessarily be related to intrinsic problems of the joint. The talocalcaneal joint may want to accommodate deformities that are more proximal (ie, at the ankle). Therefore, correction of the latter may be sufficient to unload the subtalar joint and resolve the symptoms.

REFERENCES

1. Amendola A, Lammens P. Subtalar arthrodesis using interposition iliac crest bone graft after calcaneal fracture. Foot Ankle Int 1996;17:608–14.
2. Dahm DL, Kitaoka HB. Subtalar arthrodesis with internal compression for post-traumatic arthritis. J Bone Joint Surg Br 1998;80(1):134–8.
3. Buch BD, Myerson MS, Miller SD. Primary subtalar arthrodesis for the treatment of comminuted calcaneal fractures. Foot Ankle Int 1996;17:61–70.
4. Mann RA, Beaman DN, Horton GA. Isolated subtalar arthrodesis. Foot Ankle Int 1998;19:511–9.
5. Mann RA, Baumgarten M. Subtalar fusion for isolated subtalar disorders. Preliminary report. Clin Orthop Relat Res 1988;(226):260–5.
6. Kitaoka HB, Patzer GL. Subtalar arthrodesis for posterior tibial tendon dysfunction and pes planus. Clin Orthop Relat Res 1997;(345):187–94.
7. Myerson MS. Adult acquired flatfoot deformity. Treatment of dysfunction of the posterior tibial tendon. Instr Course Lect 1997;46:393–405.
8. Boone DW. Complications of iliac crest graft and bone grafting alternatives in foot and ankle surgery. Foot Ankle Clin 2003;8:1–14.

9. Chou LB, Mann RA, Coughlin MJ, et al. Stress fracture as a complication of autogenous bone graft harvest from the distal tibia. Foot Ankle Int 2007;28: 199–201.
10. Easley ME, Trnka HJ, Schon LC, et al. Isolated subtalar arthrodesis. J Bone Joint Surg Am 2000;82(5):613–24.

Medial Approach to the Subtalar Joint
Anatomy, Indications, Technique Tips

Markus Knupp, MD*, Lukas Zwicky, MSc, Tamara Horn Lang, PhD,
Julian Röhm, MD, Beat Hintermann, MD

KEYWORDS

• Triple arthrodesis • Diple arthrodesis • Subtalar joint • Subtalar arthrodesis
• Flatfoot deformity • Posterior tibial tendon dysfunction

KEY POINTS

- The medial approach to the subtalar joint allows good visualization of the articular surfaces.
- Advantages compared with the lateral approach are found particularly in flatfoot correction, because the single-incision technique can be used in corrective fusions of rigid flatfoot deformity.
- Avascular necrosis of the talus is a rare but serious complication, and the risk can probably be avoided by avoiding posterolateral screw placement in the talar dome.

INTRODUCTION

The subtalar (ST) joint can be exposed through a lateral, a medial, or a posterior approach. The medial approach to the ST joint has mainly been popularized in corrective fusions of the hindfoot in tibialis posterior tendon dysfunction. In these cases it is frequently combined with soft tissue reconstruction medially (eg, revision of the tibialis posterior tendon or a flexor tendon transfer), additional osteotomies (such as a Cotton osteotomy), or fusions (talonavicular [TN], naviculocuneiform, tarsometatarsal joints) of the medial column.

SURGICAL ANATOMY

The ST joint consists of 3 articulating facets. Large variations of the morphology and the orientation of these surfaces have been described in cadaveric and radiological

Disclosures: The authors have nothing to disclose.
Department of Orthopaedic Surgery, Kantonsspital Baselland, Liestal, Switzerland
* Corresponding author. Department of Orthopaedic Surgery, Kantonsspital Baselland, Rheinstrasse 26, Liestal CH-4410, Switzerland.
E-mail address: markus.knupp@ksbl.ch

studies. The main force transmitter is the posterior facet. Therefore, knowledge of the shape and the orientation of this portion is crucial when planning and performing surgical procedures at the ST joint. In a weight-bearing computed tomography (CT) examination, 88% of the patients had a concave shape of the posterior facet and most patients showed a valgus orientation of the posterior facet.[1] However, some patients presented with a varus-oriented posterior facet or a flat surface as opposed to a concave shape.[1] Preoperative MRI or CT scans may therefore be helpful to determine which approach best exposes the articulating surfaces.

Combined fusions of the ST joint, the TN, and even the calcaneocuboid joint are possible through the medial approach.[2–6] Jeng and colleagues[3] showed in a cadaveric study that the medial approach allows preparation of 91% of the TN, 91% of the ST, and 90% of the calcaneocuboid joint. This finding is comparable to the lateral approach, which allows removal of 80% of the cartilage of the ST joint.[7]

The medial approach is located closer to the main neurovascular structures than the lateral incision. However, a cadaveric study that used the medial incision to perform diple (ST and TN) arthrodesis found a mean safe distance of more than 2 cm between the middle facet of the ST joint and the inferiorly located neurovascular bundle.[8]

INDICATIONS/CONTRAINDICATIONS

The medial approach to the ST joint can be used to perform open fusions, resection of coalitions, and reduction/internal fixation of calcaneal fractures. The indications and the technique for ST fusions are presented here.

Indications

Indications for fusions of the ST joint include deformity correction and treatment of degenerative joint diseases. The most common indications include arthritis of the hindfoot (rheumatoid or posttraumatic),[9–11] end-stage posterior tibial tendon dysfunction,[12–14] and neuromuscular disease–mediated hindfoot deformities.[15,16]

The authors use the medial approach for all ST fusions that are combined with TN and/or other fusions of the medial column. Most of the isolated ST joint fusions are performed through a lateral approach.

Tibialis Posterior Tendon Dysfunction

The benefits of the medial approach have mainly been described in flatfoot correction. Using a single medial approach for the traditional triple and the diple arthrodesis reduces the risk of wound healing problems, particularly in patients with severe deformities.[2,4,17–20] Furthermore, placing the incision medially has been shown to improve visualization and exposure of the transverse tarsal joint[3,4,20] and to allow good control of the position of the joints to be fused.[3,4,17,20,21] The improved visualization facilitates debridement of the joints without placing the posteromedial structures, especially the flexor hallucis longus tendon, at risk.[4,17] As an alternative to the triple arthrodesis, the ST joint can be fused in combination with the naviculocuneiform joint.[22] This procedure is done through an isolated medial approach and is indicated in flatfoot deformity with the main deformity located at the level of the ST and the naviculocuneiform joint lines.

Contraindications

ST distraction arthrodesis is performed through a posterior or a lateral approach because introduction of a bone block from a medial approach is very difficult. The lateral approach is also preferred in patients with a severe cavovarus deformity in which the ST joint cannot be visualized properly from the medial side.

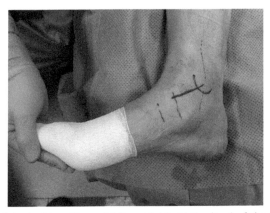

Fig. 1. Location of the incision. The solid lines highlight the level of the medial malleolus, the TN joint, and the naviculocuneiform joint. The dotted line marks the center of the medial malleolus.

SURGICAL TECHNIQUE/PROCEDURE
Preoperative Planning

Preoperative planning includes a detailed history, a thorough clinical examination, and review of the radiographs. Weight-bearing plain radiographs of the foot in the dorsoplantar and lateral projections, as well as mortise views of the ankle, are indispensable. Before surgery, arthritic degeneration of the involved joints (and of the ankle and midfoot), global bone density, and/or intraosseous cysts must be taken into consideration.

Preparation and Patient Positioning

The patient is placed in a supine position with the heel of the foot at the edge of the table. The limb is then exsanguinated and the thigh tourniquet inflated.

Surgical Procedure

Step 1
A 4-cm long skin incision is made from the medial malleolus toward the navicular, parallel to and approximately 5 mm above the tibialis posterior tendon. If the TN and/or the naviculocuneiform joints are to be exposed, the incision is extended distally (**Fig 1**).

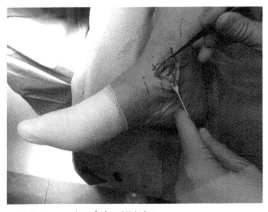

Fig. 2. The thickened joint capsule of the ST joint.

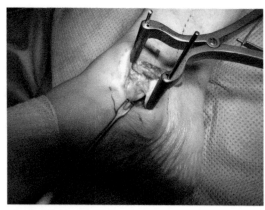

Fig. 3. Placement of the K-wire spreader: one in the talar neck and a second in the sustentaculum.

Step 2
The joint capsule is then incised (**Fig. 2**). The medial calcaneal wall is exposed down to the sustentaculum. A Kirschner wire (K-wire) is inserted into the base of the sustentaculum and a second K-wire is inserted into the talar neck. The ST joint is then distracted with a K-wire spreader (**Fig. 3**).

Step 3
Taking care not to damage the anterior fibers of the deltoid ligament, the ST joint is opened. All deep dissection remains anterior to the center of the medial malleolus (**Fig. 4**). The joint surfaces are denuded with a chisel and a curette and then feathered or drilled with a 2.0-mm drill bit.

Step 4
The foot is held in a neutral position; 2 K-wires are used to secure the position (**Figs. 5** and **6**). Stable fixation is achieved by 1 or 2 cannulated compression screws.

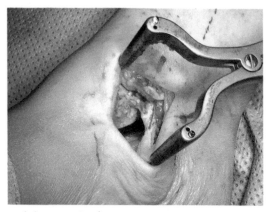

Fig. 4. The middle and the posterior facets.

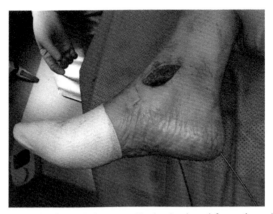

Fig. 5. K-wire placement in the ST joint: one K-wire is placed from the calcaneal tuberosity into the talar dome, the second into the talar neck.

Step 5

The joint capsule is closed with no. 0 absorbable sutures and the subcutaneous tissues and the skin are closed with interrupted sutures.

Postoperative Protocol

A compressive dressing and splint are applied and carried for 3 to 5 days. A short leg weight-bearing cast is used for 8 weeks. A rehabilitation program for strengthening, gait training, and range of motion is initiated 8 weeks after surgery, with a gradual return to full activities as tolerated.

RESULTS

In a cadaveric study the medial approach has been linked to a higher risk of decreased blood supply to the talus.[8,23] However, the published results show similar fusion rates compared with the traditional lateral approach. In our own patient cohort we observed 3 patients with avascular necrosis (AVN) in 97 ST joint fusions. One of them remained asymptomatic. In all 3 cases the screws in the talar dome were placed very far

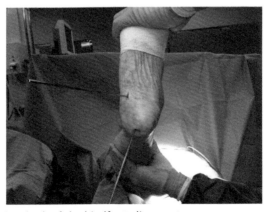

Fig. 6. Intraoperative check of the hindfoot alignment.

posterolateral. We therefore recommend placing the screws central or slightly medial and not too far posterior in the talar dome.

Anand and colleagues[5] found a nonunion in the ST joint in 1 of 18 feet (6%) that were treated with an ST and TN joint fusion through a medial incision. This finding is similar to our observation (7% in 97 feet).

Another concern with the medial approach is the potential of weakening the deltoid ligament. In a comparative study between the traditional triple arthrodesis and the diple arthrodesis, Hyer and colleagues[24] found no increased risk for deltoid ligament insufficiency in the latter group. This finding is in accordance with our observations.

A clinical example is shown in **Fig. 7**.

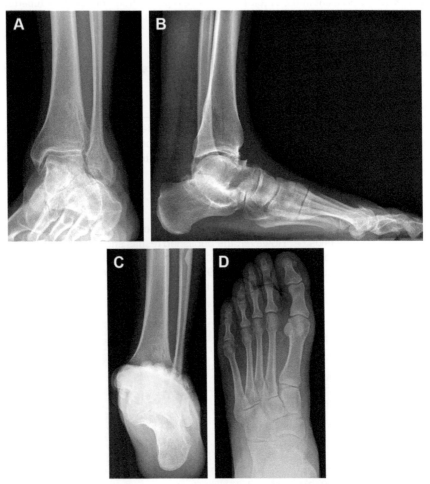

Fig. 7. A 45-year-old male patient with symptomatic ST joint arthritis and valgus malalignment of the hindfoot. (A–D) The preoperative radiographs and (E–H) the radiographs 6 months after ST joint fusion, medial displacement calcaneus osteotomy, and talar neck plasty.

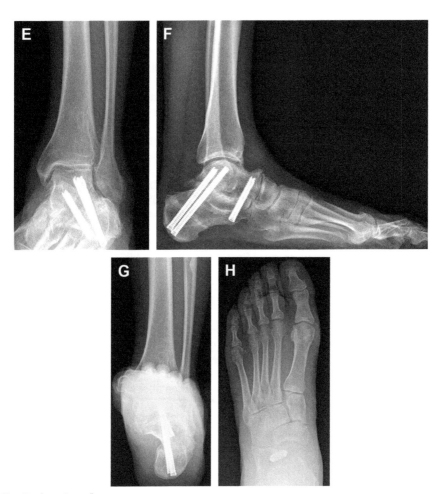

Fig. 7. (*continued*)

SUMMARY

The medial approach to the ST joint allows good visualization of the articular surfaces. Advantages compared with the lateral approach are found particularly in flatfoot correction, because the single-incision technique can be used in corrective fusions of rigid flatfoot deformity. Union rates are comparable with the traditional lateral approach and wound healing problems occur less frequently. AVN of the talus is a rare but serious complication. The risk probably can be avoided by avoiding postero-lateral screw placement in the talar dome. Earlier cadaveric studies suggested an increased risk for damage of the blood supply to the talus and to the deltoid ligament. However, clinical studies showed no increased morbidity when comparing the medial with the lateral approach.

REFERENCES

1. Colin F, Horn Lang T, Zwicky L, et al. Subtalar joint configuration on weightbearing CT scan. Foot Ankle Int 2014;35:1057–62.

2. Jeng CL, Vora AM, Myerson MS. The medial approach to triple arthrodesis. Indications and technique for management of rigid valgus deformities in high-risk patients. Foot Ankle Clin 2005;10(3):515–21, vi–vii.

3. Jeng CL, Tankson CJ, Myerson MS. The single medial approach to triple arthrodesis: a cadaver study. Foot Ankle Int 2006;27(12):1122–5.

4. Knupp M, Schuh R, Stufkens SA, et al. Subtalar and talonavicular arthrodesis through a single medial approach for the correction of severe planovalgus deformity. J Bone Joint Surg Br 2009;91(5):612–5.

5. Anand P, Nunley JA, Deorio JK. Single-incision medial approach for double arthrodesis of hindfoot in posterior tibialis tendon dysfunction. Foot Ankle Int 2013;34(3):338–44.

6. Brilhault J. Single medial approach to modified double arthrodesis in rigid flatfoot with lateral deficient skin. Foot Ankle Int 2009;30(1):21–6.

7. Bono JV, Jacobs RL. Triple arthrodesis through a single lateral approach: a cadaveric experiment. Foot Ankle 1992;13(7):408–12.

8. Galli MM, Scott RT, Bussewitz B, et al. Structures at risk with medial double hindfoot fusion: a cadaveric study. J Foot Ankle Surg 2014;53:598–600.

9. Figgie MP, O'Malley MJ, Ranawat C, et al. Triple arthrodesis in rheumatoid arthritis. Clin Orthop Relat Res 1993;(292):250–4.

10. Knupp M, Skoog A, Tornkvist H, et al. Triple arthrodesis in rheumatoid arthritis. Foot Ankle Int 2008;29(3):293–7.

11. Klaue K. Chopart fractures. Injury 2004;35(Suppl 2):SB64–70.

12. Saltzman CL, Fehrle MJ, Cooper RR, et al. Triple arthrodesis: twenty-five and forty-four-year average follow-up of the same patients. J Bone Joint Surg Am 1999;81(10):1391–402.

13. Pell RF, Myerson MS, Schon LC. Clinical outcome after primary triple arthrodesis. J Bone Joint Surg Am 2000;82(1):47–57.

14. Bennett GL, Graham CE, Mauldin DM. Triple arthrodesis in adults. Foot Ankle 1991;12(3):138–43.

15. The classic. Arthrodesing operations on the feet: Edwin W. Ryerson, M. D. Clin Orthop Relat Res 1977;(122):4–9.

16. Wetmore RS, Drennan JC. Long-term results of triple arthrodesis in Charcot-Marie-Tooth disease. J Bone Joint Surg Am 1989;71(3):417–22.

17. DeWachter J, Knupp M, Hintermann B. Double-hindfoot arthrodesis through a single medial approach. Tech Foot Ankle Surg 2007;6(4):237–42.

18. Jackson WF, Tryfonidis M, Cooke PH, et al. Arthrodesis of the hindfoot for valgus deformity. An entirely medial approach. J Bone Joint Surg Br 2007;89(7):925–7.

19. Knupp M, Stufkens SA, Hintermann B. Triple arthrodesis. Foot Ankle Clin 2011; 16(1):61–7.

20. Saville P, Longman CF, Srinivasan SC, et al. Medial approach for hindfoot arthrodesis with a valgus deformity. Foot Ankle Int 2011;32(8):818–21.

21. Catanzariti AR, Adeleke AT. Double arthrodesis through a medial approach for end-stage adult-acquired flatfoot. Clin Podiatr Med Surg 2014;31(3):435–44.

22. Gilgen A, Knupp M, Hintermann B. Subtalar and naviculo-cuneiform arthrodesis for treatment of hindfoot valgus with collapse of the medial arch. Tech Foot Ankle Surg 2013;12(4):190–5.

23. Phisitkul P, Haugsdal J, Vaseenon T, et al. Vascular disruption of the talus: comparison of two approaches for triple arthrodesis. Foot Ankle Int 2013;34(4):568–74.

24. Hyer CF, Galli MM, Scott RT, et al. Ankle valgus after hindfoot arthrodesis: a radiographic and chart comparison of the medial double and triple arthrodeses. J Foot Ankle Surg 2014;53(1):55–8.

Subtalar Joint Arthrodesis

Open and Arthroscopic Indications and Surgical Techniques

Brent Roster, MD*, Christopher Kreulen, MD, Eric Giza, MD

KEYWORDS

• Arthrodesis • Subtalar • Joint • Arthroscopy • Hindfoot

KEY POINTS

• Both arthroscopic and open subtalar joint arthrodesis techniques can successfully be used to treat conditions causing pain, deformity, or both.
• High fusion rates and functional improvement have been reported after both open and arthroscopic arthrodesis.
• Posterior and lateral arthroscopy of the subtalar joint have been shown to have few complications and high fusion rates.
• Arthroscopic subtalar fusion may be associated with higher fusion rates, shorter hospital stays, and fewer complications relative to open procedures; however, the two need to be compared further in order to definitively make that assertion.

BACKGROUND/ANATOMY

The talocalcaneal joint is formed by a combination of 3 articulating surfaces: the anterior, middle, and posterior facets. Its unique composition and the orientation of its facets allows for motion in 3 planes: inversion/eversion, flexion/extension, and abduction/adduction.[1] This triaxial motion, in combination with the plantar flexion/dorsiflexion of the tibiotalar joint, is critical for ambulation on uneven ground.[1,2] The primary arc of motion of the subtalar joint is inversion/supination (25°–30°) and eversion/pronation (5°–10°) (**Fig. 1**).[1,3]

The subtalar joint is also critical for normal foot mechanics and ambulation. With the subtalar joint everted, or in valgus, the transverse tarsal joints are unlocked, which allows a smooth transition from heel strike to stance phase. As gait progresses through stance phase, the hindfoot inverts; this locks the transverse tarsal joints,

Disclosure: Dr B. Roster and Dr C. Kreulen have nothing to disclose. Dr E. Giza is the consultant for Arthrex and Zimmer.
UC Davis Medical Center, Sacramento, Department of Orthopaedic Surgery, 4860 Y Street, Suite 3800, Sacramento, CA 95817, USA
* Corresponding author. Reno Orthopaedic Clinic, 555 N. Arlington Avenue, Reno, NV 89503.
E-mail address: brentroster@gmail.com

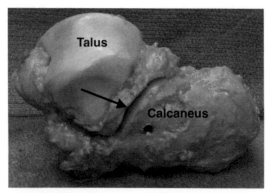

Fig. 1. Gross specimen of a talus and calcaneus (*left*) showing their relationship, as viewed from the lateral side. The arrow is pointing to the posterior facet.

providing a rigid lever and allowing propulsion forward.[4] The biomechanics of the subtalar joint are therefore crucial to understanding correct and appropriate positioning of the subtalar joint when performing an arthrodesis.

SUBTALAR JOINT DISORDERS AND HINDFOOT DEFORMITY

Many different types of disorder can affect the subtalar joint and lead to pain, deformity, or both. These disorders include primary osteoarthritis, congenital conditions, inflammatory arthropathies, postseptic arthritis, posttraumatic arthritis, acquired conditions such as adult acquired flatfoot deformity, and chronic subtalar joint instability refractory to conservative treatments or reconstructive procedures (**Box 1**).[1–3,5–14] Subtalar arthrodesis can be used successfully to treat all of these conditions, with the goal of

---

Box 1
Conditions affecting the subtalar joint

Primary osteoarthritis

Inflammatory arthropathy

   Rheumatoid arthritis

Congenital conditions

   Talocalcaneal coalitions

   Neuromuscular disorders (eg, cerebral palsy)

Postseptic arthritis

Posttraumatic arthritis

   Calcaneus fracture

   Talus fracture

   Subtalar dislocation

Acquired conditions

   Adult acquired flatfoot deformity

   Postpolio syndrome

Chronic subtalar joint instability

relieving pain; improving the patients' function; and providing them with a stable, plantigrade foot.

WORK-UP/EVALUATION

Work-up of patients with hindfoot disorders begins with a thorough history and physical examination. Patients with subtalar joint disease often complain of lateral ankle pain, difficulty walking on uneven ground, and of pain localized around the sinus tarsi, especially with hindfoot inversion and eversion. Physical examination reveals lateral hindfoot swelling, pain with subtalar joint range of motion, and tenderness in the sinus tarsi. The patient's gait should be observed. Subtalar motion should be tested and compared with the contralateral side; pain with inversion and eversion of the hindfoot with ankle held in neutral dorsiflexion suggests a subtalar joint disorder. Other potential sources of pain should be investigated and ruled out.

Imaging includes standing anteroposterior (AP), lateral, and oblique views of the foot; standing AP, lateral, and mortise views of the ankle; and hindfoot alignment views. Additional radiographs can be obtained, including a Harris heel view, Broden view (visualizes the posterior facet of the talocalcaneal joint), and Canale view (visualizes the sinus tarsi). Computed tomography (CT) should be performed on most patients, because it can be helpful in evaluating the extent of arthrosis and deformity as well as identifying the presence of a coalition (**Fig. 2**).

Once the subtalar joint has been identified as the source of a patient's pain, a diagnostic injection can be helpful in confirming the diagnosis, and may provide the patient with short-term or long-term relief.

TREATMENT
Nonoperative Treatment

Nonoperative treatment of subtalar joint disorder begins with activity modification. In some conditions, such as chronic subtalar joint instability, physical therapy focusing on proprioception and peroneal strengthening may be of benefit.[1,3] High-top shoes, bracing, and orthotics can sometimes be helpful, although bracing of the subtalar joint is difficult and is best accomplished with a semirigid or rigid ankle-foot orthosis.[3]

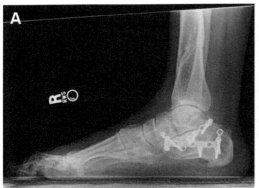
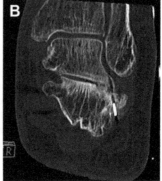

Fig. 2. Posttraumatic arthritis of the subtalar joint in a patient 15 years status post calcaneus fracture and open reduction with internal fixation, ultimately treated with hardware removal and open subtalar joint fusion using a sinus tarsi approach. (*A*) Standing lateral radiograph of the foot. (*B*) Representative coronal slice from the patient's CT scan showing advanced degeneration of the posterior facet.

Orthotics are commonly used to address hindfoot malalignment. Subtalar joint injections can be of benefit to patients who wish to avoid surgery. In addition, antiinflammatories should be trialed if there are no contraindications to their use.

Operative Treatment: Subtalar Arthrodesis

If nonoperative treatment fails, arthrodesis can be considered. The goals of hindfoot arthrodesis include pain relief, deformity correction, and functional improvement by providing the patient with a stable, plantigrade foot.[2,15] Because the subtalar joint plays a vital role in foot and gait biomechanics, great attention must be paid to the position of the arthrodesis. A biomechanical study performed by Jastifer and colleagues[16] evaluated various positions of subtalar arthrodesis in a computational lower extremity model with regard to dorsiflexion and plantar flexion strength, moments, and moment arms through a physiologic range of motion; plantar flexion strength was maximized at an arthrodesis position of 10° of valgus, and dorsiflexion strength maximized at 5° of valgus. Their study thus supported the general consensus that fusing the subtalar joint in 5° to 10° of valgus is optimal biomechanically.

Many different techniques for subtalar fusion have been described, and these vary in surgical approach, implant choices, number and orientation of screws, and so forth. Despite this variability, several general principles, as described by Mann and numerous others, should be followed to ensure the best possible outcome and avoid complications such as wound breakdown, nonunion, or malunion[2,15,17]:

- Incisions should be thoughtfully planned and the soft tissues should be handled with care.
- Joint preparation should be thorough and meticulous, and broad, congruent, bleeding cancellous surfaces should be created, ideally so that apposition of those surfaces can be obtained. All articular cartilage should be removed, as should the subchondral bone.
- Fixation of the arthrodesis site should be rigid.
- Particular attention should be paid to the position and alignment of the arthrodesis, as outlined earlier.

INDICATIONS AND TECHNIQUES OF SUBTALAR ARTHRODESIS
Open Subtalar Arthrodesis

Traditional or open subtalar joint arthrodesis and its outcomes have been extensively reported in the literature. As noted earlier, many different techniques have been described.[2,5–10,15,17]

Indications and contraindications

Open subtalar joint arthrodesis can be performed for any of the primary arthritic, posttraumatic, congenital, or neuromuscular disorders listed earlier. In general, an open approach to subtalar joint arthrodesis is preferred for conditions involving large hindfoot deformity or malalignment, significant bone loss of the talus or calcaneus, prior subtalar joint nonunion or malunion, and cases requiring large bone grafting.[2,6–10,15–18] Open subtalar joint arthrodesis is particularly useful in treatment of calcaneus fracture malunion; in addition to posttraumatic arthritis caused by articular cartilage injury, these injuries often heal with loss of calcaneal height, varus, heel widening with subsequent calcaneal-fibular impingement and peroneal tendon and sural nerve irritation, anterior ankle impingement caused by loss of normal talus declination, and calcaneal-cuboid joint impingement.[5,9] Surgical techniques to address these sequelae that are not possible with an isolated arthroscopic approach include decompression of the lateral wall of the calcaneus, distraction bone-block arthrodesis of the subtalar joint to restore calcaneal height, bone grafting to address large amounts of bone loss, and corrective osteotomies, all of which can be performed in concert with an open subtalar arthrodesis (**Fig. 3**).[5,7,10] In short, an open subtalar arthrodesis may be chosen when a larger exposure is needed for additional procedures in addition to fusion of the talocalcaneal joint.

Contraindications to open subtalar joint arthrodesis include tenuous skin or compromised soft tissue envelope in the area of planned incisions, patients in whom wound healing is a concern, and active infection.

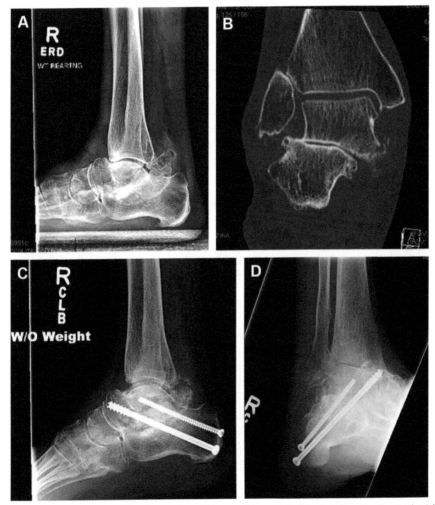

Fig. 3. A patient with a talocalcaneal coalition and large hindfoot deformity, treated with distraction bone-block subtalar arthrodesis. (*A*) Standing lateral radiograph of the foot showing hindfoot valgus, anterior impingement, and effective loss of calcaneal height, with large posterior osteophyte. (*B*) Representative coronal CT slice showing subluxation of the posterior facet and associated degenerative changes. (*C, D*) Postoperative radiographs showing fusion of the subtalar joint with restoration of calcaneal height.

Technique

The following is the senior author's preferred technique for open subtalar arthrodesis:

- Positioning and setup:
  - The patient is given appropriate preoperative antibiotics.
  - General and regional anesthesia (popliteal block) are used.
  - A tourniquet is placed on the upper thigh.
  - The patient is positioned in the lateral decubitus position on a bean bag, with care taken to pad the nonoperative leg and axilla. A level platform is built out of folded blankets for the operative leg to rest on (**Fig. 4**A).
- Approach and exposure:
  - Bony landmarks are marked out on the skin with a marker, and a curvilinear incision is marked out from the distal aspect of the fibula down toward the base of the fourth metatarsal.
  - The skin is incised with a 15-blade scalpel. Electrocautery is used to go through crossing veins.
  - The extensor digitorum brevis is then encountered; this is carefully elevated with a distally based flap/pedicle so as to preserve its blood supply.
  - The peroneal tendons are retracted posteriorly and distally.
  - Access to the sinus tarsi is then possible. A rongeur is used to remove the fat from this area. At this point, the interosseous talocalcaneal ligament is visible and should be removed to allow greater distraction and visualization of the joint.

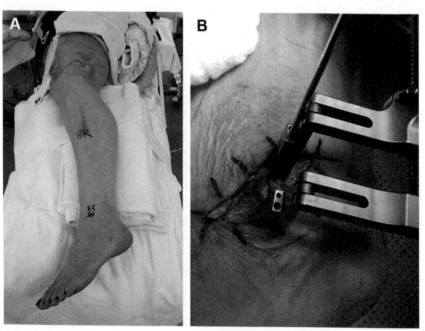

Fig. 4. (*A*) Positioning of the patient for open subtalar joint fusion. The patient is positioned laterally on a bean bag with the foot at the end of the bed, and a stack of blankets is built up under the operative leg, stopping short of the foot (this allows for easier screw placement after joint preparation). (*B*) Open subtalar joint arthrodesis using a sinus tarsi approach; a commercially available distractor using K-wires is used for distraction of the joint.

- o The dissection can then be taken distally and the talonavicular capsule and joint are easily identified.
  - o The subtalar joint can then be entered and distracted. A lamina spreader or distractor using Kirschner wires (K-wires) can be used (see **Fig. 4**B).
- Joint preparation:
  - o All articular cartilage of the posterior and middle facets must be removed. The soft tissue and the cortical bone of the sinus tarsi should also be removed, creating a greater surface area for fusion, which is accomplished with a combination of curettes and the use of an osteotome to remove the subchondral bone.
  - o The joint is then thoroughly irrigated.
  - o A drill is then used to penetrate the bony surfaces down to bleeding bone. Next, an osteotome is used to fish scale the bony surfaces to increase the surface area available for fusion. Once these steps are completed, a slurry should be present in the joint.
  - o Bone graft can then be harvested from the calcaneus using a commercially available bone graft harvester. The starting point is on the lateral calcaneus, and the harvester is directed anteriorly and superiorly.
  - o This harvested bone graft is then mixed with demineralized bone matrix and placed into the posterior and middle facets.
  - o Distraction is then removed, and the subtalar joint is compressed and manually held in 5° to 7° of valgus.
- Screw placement
  - o Fixation is provided by 2 partially threaded large-fragment cannulated screws placed across the subtalar joint:
  - o Two K-wires are placed through the heel, proximal to the weight-bearing surface. One is directed across the joint into the talar neck and its placement is verified on lateral, Broden, and AP foot views, as well as a Harris heel view to ensure that the medial calcaneus has not been penetrated. A second K-wire is placed parallel in the sagittal plane, superior to the first, and is placed in a divergent manner up into the subchondral bone of the talar dome. The wires are then measured and the screw holes drilled.
  - o Two 6.7-mm screws are then placed. Stab incisions are made along the K-wires and blunt dissection made down to bone. As the first screw is being placed, the other wire is brought back across the joint so as to achieve maximum compression across the joint with the first screw. The second screw is then placed and their positions are checked with fluoroscopy (AP, lateral, Broden, and Harris heel views).
  - o If additional lateral compression is desired, a 15 × 15 mm staple can be placed through drill holes in the lateral process of the talus and the lateral calcaneus. If this is done, the clinician must be sure to check that there is no impingement of the distal fibula on the staple.
  - o Thorough irrigation of the incisions is then performed. Additional bone graft is packed into the sinus tarsi, and the extensor digitorum brevis and subcutaneous tissues are closed with 3-0 Vicryl suture. The tourniquet is then let down and hemostasis is obtained. The skin is then closed with 3-0 nylon suture. A sterile dressing is then applied, followed by a well-padded short leg splint.

Postoperative care

- Weeks 0 to 2: the patient is immobilized and kept non–weight bearing in a short leg splint. The wounds are checked at 10 to 14 days and the sutures removed.

- Weeks 3 to 6: the patient is placed in a removable boot for the daytime, and a removable night splint for sleeping. The patient is kept non–weight bearing. At 6 weeks, the patient is seen in the office and radiographs are obtained (AP, lateral, and mortise views of the ankle). Some clinicians prefer to use a short leg cast during this period.
- Weeks 7 to 12: as long as adequate healing is suspected at the 6-week postoperative visit, the patient is allowed to begin progressive partial weight bearing in a boot. Physical therapy is started after the 6-week visit. The patient is seen in clinic again at 12 weeks after surgery, and repeat radiographs are obtained. If solid fusion is noted, full weight bearing is allowed out of the boot.

Arthroscopic Subtalar Arthrodesis

Arthroscopy of the subtalar joint was first described in 1985 by Parisien and Vangness,[19] and has since evolved and its indications expanded.[20–23] Arthroscopic subtalar arthrodesis was first reported in the literature in 1994 by Lundeen[24] and by Tasto at the Arthroscopic Association of North America's annual meeting, also in 1994.[13] Performing this procedure arthroscopically is appealing in its potential advantages compared with open arthrodesis given its smaller incisions, theoretic preservation of calcaneal and talar blood supply, less damage to the soft tissue envelope, and less perioperative morbidity.[12–14,20]

Arthroscopic portals for the subtalar joint can be placed laterally, posteriorly, or both. For lateral arthroscopy of the subtalar joint, the patient is placed in either a supine or lateral position. Several portals have been described, including anterolateral, posterolateral, accessory anterolateral and accessory posterolateral, and central portals.[14,20,22,23] Either the 30° 2.7-mm or 1.9-mm arthroscope may be used, depending on the amount of distraction obtained. If needed for visualization, the 70° arthroscope can be used as well. Traction is useful in improving visualization of the joint. With arthroscopic subtalar arthrodesis, the posterior facet articulation is prepared using a combination of curettes, burrs, osteotomes, and awls. With lateral subtalar arthroscopy, it has been shown cadaverically that 90% of the posterior facet can be resected using just the central and anterolateral portals, thereby avoiding the posterolateral portal and the potential for sural nerve and small saphenous vein injury.[20]

Posterior subtalar arthroscopy offers an alternative to lateral-based arthroscopy, and is performed in the prone position. Proponents of posterior subtalar joint arthroscopy cite improved visualization of the coronal alignment of the hindfoot and subtalar joint (because of prone positioning) and avoidance of damage to the vessels of the sinus tarsi (and thus preserving more talar blood supply) as benefits compared with using strictly laterally based portals.[21,25–28] Phisitkul and colleagues[26] reported on the working area of posterior subtalar joint arthroscopy in cadavers; using posterolateral and posteromedial portals (both adjacent to the Achilles tendon), without the use of distraction or an irrigation pump, the combination of these two posterior portals provided a working area of 43% of this articulation. However, they defined this working area as the amount of the articular surface that could be accessed without damaging the articular cartilage; thus, by removing cartilage as in the case of an arthrodesis, visualization and working area should be increased. As reported by Beals and colleagues,[27] the use of traction for distraction can improve posterior arthroscopic access to the joint as well. Potential dangers of posterior subtalar joint arthroscopy include damage to the peroneal tendons (posterolateral portal) and damage to the posterior tibial neurovascular bundle and medical calcaneal nerve (posteromedial portal) (**Fig. 5**).[28]

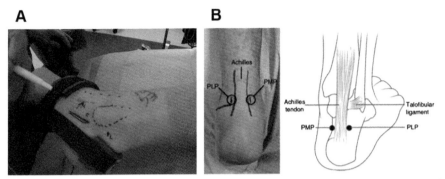

Fig. 5. Portal location for lateral and posterior subtalar joint arthroscopy. (*A*) Location of lateral portals (left foot) with associated anatomic structures at risk drawn out on the skin. A noninvasive distraction strap is in place. The fibula is marked out (*dotted line*), as are the superficial peroneal nerve (*solid line*) and the course of the peroneal tendons (*double solid line* inferior to the fibula). The course of the sural nerve is not drawn out. (*B*) Posterior portal location. AL, anterolateral portal; C, central portal; PL, posterolateral portal; PLP, posterolateral portal; PMP, posteromedial portal. (*From* Hsu AR, Gross CE, Lee S, et al. Extended indications for foot and ankle arthroscopy. J Am Acad Orthop Surg 2014;22:11; with permission).

Indications and contraindications

Arthroscopic subtalar arthrodesis can be performed for the same indications as those discussed with open procedures, with the exception of large deformities, bone loss, previous nonunion or malunion requiring large dissection or large amounts of bone graft, and in patients in whom access to the subtalar joint is not thought to be possible using arthroscopy and noninvasive or minimally invasive distraction techniques. Arthroscopic arthrodesis is also an attractive approach for patients with wound healing concerns, compromised soft tissues, or who have had previous surgeries in the area of a planned open incision.

Technique

The following is the senior author's preferred technique for arthroscopic subtalar arthrodesis:

- Patient positioning/setup (**Fig. 6**A)
  - The patient is given appropriate preoperative antibiotics after receiving a popliteal block in the preoperative holding area, and is placed under general anesthesia.
  - A tourniquet is placed around the upper thigh. The patient is then placed in the lateral decubitus position, with care taken to pad the nonoperative leg and axilla.
  - The operative leg is placed in an arthroscopic leg holder with gel pads for protection. The patient's operative foot should not be at the end of the bed, but at least 30 to 50 cm toward the head of the bed to allow for proper traction setup and maintenance.
  - The operative leg is then prepped and draped in the standard sterile manner.
  - A transcalcaneal traction pin (5.0-mm centrally threaded Steinmann pin) is placed from medial to lateral. Care must be taken to keep this in the inferior-posterior aspect of the calcaneus so as not to interfere with manipulation/use of arthroscopic instruments. From 5.5 to 9 kg (12–20 pounds) of traction are hung over an extension at the end of the bed (see **Fig. 6**B).

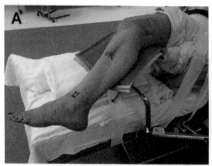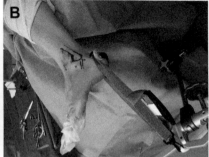

Fig. 6. (A) Patient positioning for lateral subtalar joint arthroscopy. The patient is lateral on a bean bag, with the operative leg placed on an arthroscopic leg holder. (B) Transcalcaneal traction setup.

- Portal placement:
  - The central portal for access to the subtalar joint is first placed under fluoroscopic guidance. The location of this portal is approximately 1 cm anterior and 1 cm distal to the tip of the fibula. An 18-gauge spinal needle is directed into the subtalar joint, and 10 mL of fluid are injected to distend the joint. A 15-blade scalpel is used to incise the skin, with blunt dissection down to and through the joint capsule. The cannula is then introduced into the subtalar joint, followed by the 1.9-mm or 2.7-mm arthroscope. The peroneal tendons and the sural nerve can be at risk in placing this portal, so care must be taken (**Fig. 7**A, B).
  - The posterior-lateral portal is established next. An 18-gauge needle is placed through the skin at a location approximately halfway between the Achilles tendon and the posterior border of the fibula, at about the level of the tip of the fibula. This portal is established under direct visualization, with the arthroscope in the central portal. A 15-blade scalpel is used to incise the skin. Care must be taken to longitudinally dissect through the soft tissues in order to prevent injury to the sural nerve (see **Fig. 7**C).
  - The shaver can then be introduced into the posterolateral portal, and any synovitis can be removed in order to improve visualization of the joint.
  - The anterolateral portal is made last. The location of this portal is approximately 1 cm distal and 0.5 cm anterior to the central portal. Again, a 15-blade scalpel is used to incise the skin, followed by blunt dissection down to the interosseous talocalcaneal ligament. The cannula can then be introduced under direct visualization, with the arthroscope in the central portal.
  - After joint debridement with the shaver in the anterolateral portal, the interosseous talocalcaneal ligament is transected percutaneously using a 15-blade scalpel; this serves to provide further visualization of the joint.
- Joint preparation:
  - The articular surfaces of the posterior facet are then sequentially denuded using a curette and by switching viewing and working portals.
  - Fluoroscopy is used to ensure that access to the entire joint has been attained.
  - Thorough irrigation is completed, thereby removing all floating pieces of cartilage and debris.
  - A 4.5-mm burr is then used to sequentially remove all subchondral bone down to a bleeding bed, taking care to maintain the overall geometry of the joint

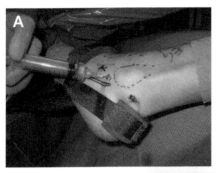

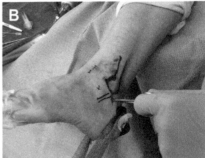

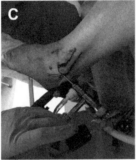

Fig. 7. Establishing lateral portals. (*A*) Injection through the location of the central portal in order to distend the subtalar joint. (*B*) Blunt dissection to the level of the capsule, central portal. (*C*) Establishment of the posterolateral portal under direct visualization using a spinal needle, with the arthroscope in the central portal.

> (unless trying to correct a deformity). Inflow is then turned off and dry arthroscopy is used to verify adequate bone bleeding (**Fig. 8**).
> - Five cubic centimeters of demineralized bone matrix putty are then placed into the joint through the central and posterolateral portals, and traction is removed. The traction pin is then removed as well.
> - Screw placement:
>   - With traction removed, the hindfoot is placed and held in approximately 5° of valgus. Position of the hindfoot is verified on AP, lateral, Broden, and Harris heel views using fluoroscopy.

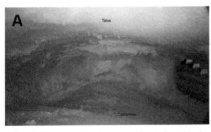

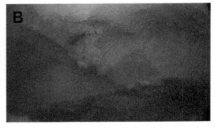

Fig. 8. Arthroscopic pictures of a left subtalar joint, with the arthroscope in the central portal. (*A*) Joint after debridement with a shaver, showing extensive articular cartilage loss. The shaver is in the posterolateral portal. (*B*) Joint surfaces after removal of subchondral bone with a burr.

- Two diverging K-wires are then placed antegrade across the subtalar joint in a similar fashion as described earlier. The inferior K-wire is driven through the calcaneus into the talar neck; the more superior K-wire is driven across the calcaneus in a similar fashion, but into the talar body. Fluoroscopy is used to ensure that both wires are within the calcaneus (Harris heel view), and they are then measured for length.
- Two 6.7-mm partially threaded cannulated screws are then advanced over the wires. Fluoroscopy is again used to ensure that the screw tips have not violated the tibiotalar or talonavicular joints. The K-wires are then removed **(Fig. 9)**.
- The portals and screw entry holes are then thoroughly irrigated. The incisions are closed in a layered fashion with 3-0 Monocryl and 3-0 nylon suture. A sterile dressing and then a well-padded short leg splint are then applied.

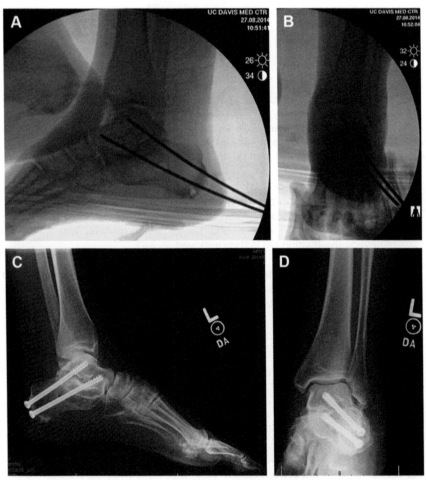

Fig. 9. (*A, B*) Intraoperative lateral and mortise views showing K-wire placement for cannulated screws. (*C, D*) Radiographs showing screw placement at the patient's first postoperative appointment.

Postoperative care

The same postoperative protocol as described earlier is followed after arthroscopic subtalar joint fusion (**Fig. 10**).

RESULTS

Both open and arthroscopic subtalar joint fusion are associated with good results; several series of both techniques have been reported in the literature. Reported fusion rates and functional outcomes from open subtalar arthrodesis are high for nearly all indications. Senaran and colleagues[6] reported on their results of subtalar fusion in 138 consecutive children with cerebral palsy; fusion rate was 96% and occurred at a mean of 6.4 weeks. Carranza-Bencano and colleagues[18] reported a fusion rate of 92% in 77 feet treated with minimal-incision subtalar arthrodesis, with good outcomes in 57 patients, fair in 13, and poor in 7. In this series, American Orthopaedic Foot and Ankle Society (AOFAS) scores had improved by a mean of 47.6 points at 12 months postoperatively. Another series of 20 patients reported an 80% fusion rate at an average of 15.75 weeks using a standard open technique.[29] Joveniaux and colleagues[30] reported on their series of 37 consecutive isolated subtalar arthrodeses, of which 23 patients were active smokers at the time of procedure; of the 28 cases not lost to follow-up, 21 had evidence of complete bony fusion at a mean of 13 weeks, and none of the patients without evidence of bony union had clinical manifestations of a nonunion. The smokers in this series achieved bony union in the same time period as the nonsmokers, and the rate of incomplete bony union of 24% in these patients was

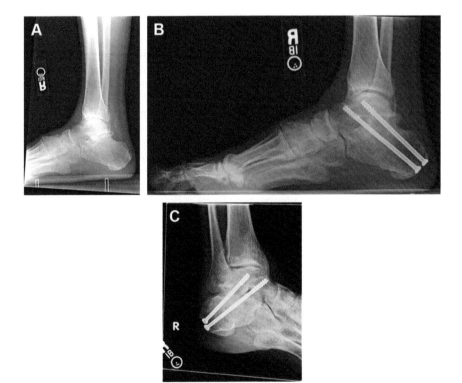

Fig. 10. Isolated symptomatic subtalar joint arthritis. (*A*) Standing lateral radiograph. (*B, C*) Postoperative imaging at 6 months showing solid bony union.

nearly the same as that of nonsmokers (29%). The investigators also noted that mild arthritic changes occurred in 12 tibiotalar, 18 talonavicular, and 15 calcaneocuboid joints with median follow-up at 56 months, although these radiographic changes did not correlate with decreased functional scores. Diezi and colleagues[31] reported a 93% union rate in 15 patients, again with significant improvement in functional scores. Several studies reporting on open subtalar arthrodesis for pes planovalgus report fusion rates of 100% without bone grafting.[8] Union rates for primary subtalar arthrodesis for severely comminuted calcaneus fractures have been reported to be between 90% and 100%.[32] Overall, the rates of nonunion reported in the literature range between 0% and 43%, with suggested risk factors of diabetes, smoking, posttraumatic arthritis, and surgical technique, although these have not been borne out in all studies.[33] Most studies of open subtalar arthrodesis report union rates of near or more than 90%.

Similarly, arthroscopic subtalar fusion rates and functional outcomes are also high. Fusion rates after arthroscopic arthrodesis reportedly range from 89% to 100%.[13] Glanzmann and Sanhueza-Hernandez[34] reported on a prospective series of 41 arthroscopic subtalar arthrodeses performed with lateral portals; the average hospital stay was 2 days, with a 100% fusion rate at a mean of 11 weeks. Three delayed unions were noted, all in patients in whom no immobilization was used. Bone grafting was done in all cases. Amendola and colleagues[28] reported on 11 cases using posterior subtalar arthroscopy; 10 of 11 joints were fused at an average of 10 weeks, with significantly improved AOFAS scores.

Few studies have compared open with arthroscopic subtalar arthrodesis. Scranton[35] reviewed results of isolated, in situ subtalar arthrodesis (8 open, 5 arthroscopic), and hospital length of stay was an average of 2.7 days in the open group and 1 night in the arthroscopic group. Average tourniquet time was slightly longer in the arthroscopic group (63 minutes vs 58 minutes). There was 1 nonunion in the open group (a diabetic patient), and none in the arthroscopic group. A systematic review performed by Stegeman and colleagues[36] reported that AOFAS scores were higher after arthroscopic subtalar arthrodesis compared with open procedures, although this may be confounded by lower AOFAS scores preoperatively in the open group. Time to bony union was also noted to be faster in the arthroscopic group (9 weeks vs 18 weeks for open procedures), and the number of reported complications lower. Improvement in AOFAS score was greater in the open arthrodesis group in this series.

Although fusion rates and functional outcome improvements are high after both open and arthroscopic arthrodeses, isolated subtalar joint arthrodesis has consequences. In the short and long terms, both types of procedures have complications, including superficial and deep infection, nonunion, malunion, neurovascular injury, complex regional pain syndrome, asymptomatic and symptomatic arthritis development in adjacent joints, and hardware prominence and failure requiring secondary procedures.[5–11,13,14,17,18,22,27,30–38]

SUMMARY

After conservative measures have failed, both arthroscopic and open subtalar joint arthrodesis techniques can successfully be used to treat conditions causing pain, deformity, or both. Each technique has its own set of indications, contraindications, and complications. High fusion rates and functional improvement have been reported after both open and arthroscopic arthrodesis. Both posterior and lateral arthroscopy of the subtalar joint have been shown to have few complications and high fusion rates. Arthroscopic subtalar fusion may be associated with higher fusion rates, shorter hospital stays, and fewer complications relative to open procedures; however, the two need to be compared further in order to definitively make that assertion.

REFERENCES

1. Keefe DT, Haddad SL. Subtalar instability: etiology, diagnosis, and management. Foot Ankle Clin N Am 2002;7:577–609.
2. Greisberg J, Sangeorzan B. Hindfoot arthrodesis. J Am Acad Orthop Surg 2007; 15(1):65–71.
3. Barg A, Tochigi Y, Amendola A, et al. Subtalar instability: diagnosis and treatment. Foot Ankle Int 2012;33:151–60.
4. Mann RA, Haskell A. Biomechanics of the foot and ankle. In: Coughlin MJ, Mann RA, Saltzman CL, editors. Surgery of the foot and ankle. 8th edition. Philadelphia: Elsevier Health; 2007. p. 3–45.
5. Banerjee R, Saltzman C, Anderson RB, et al. Management of calcaneal malunion. J Am Acad Orthop Surg 2011;19(1):27–36.
6. Senaran H, Yilmaz G, Nagai MK, et al. Subtalar fusion in cerebral palsy patients: Results of a new technique using corticocancellous allograft. J Pediatr Orthop 2001;31(2):205–10.
7. Amendola A, Lammens P. Subtalar arthrodesis using interposition iliac crest bone graft after calcaneal fracture. Foot Ankle Int 1996;17:608–14.
8. Kadakia AR, Haddad SL. Hindfoot arthrodesis for the adult acquired flat foot. Foot Ankle Clin N Am 2003;8:569–94.
9. Robinson JF, Murphy GA. Arthrodesis as salvage for calcaneal malunions. Foot Ankle Clin N Am 2002;7:107–20.
10. Molloy AP, Lipscombe SJ. Hindfoot arthrodesis for management of bone loss following calcaneus fractures and nonunions. Foot Ankle Clin N Am 2011;16: 165–79.
11. Hsu AR, Gross CE, Lee S, et al. Extended indications for foot and ankle arthroscopy. J Am Acad Orthop Surg 2014;22:10–9.
12. Narita N, Takao M, Innami K, et al. Minimally invasive subtalar arthrodesis with iliac crest autograft through posterior arthroscopic portals: a technical note. Foot Ankle Int 2012;33:803–5.
13. Stroud CC. Arthroscopic arthrodesis of the ankle, subtalar, and first metatarsophalangeal joint. Foot Ankle Clin North Am 2002;7:135–46.
14. Muraro GM, Carvajal PF. Arthroscopic arthrodesis of subtalar joint. Foot Ankle Clin N Am 2011;16:83–90.
15. Mann RA. Arthrodesis of the foot and ankle. In: Coughlin MJ, Mann RA, Saltzman CL, editors. Surgery of the foot and ankle. 8th edition. Philadelphia: Elsevier Health; 2007. p. 1087–123.
16. Jastifer JR, Gustafson PA, Gorman RR. Subtalar arthrodesis alignment: the effect on ankle biomechanics. Foot Ankle Int 2013;34:244–50.
17. Tuijthof GJ, Beimers L, Kerkhoffs GM, et al. Overview of subtalar arthrodesis techniques: Options, pitfalls, and solutions. J Foot Ankle Surg 2010;16:107–16.
18. Carranza-Bencano A, Tejero-Garcia S, Del Castillo-Blanco G, et al. Isolated subtalar arthrodesis through minimal incision surgery. Foot Ankle Int 2013;34:1117–27.
19. Parisien JS, Vangsness T. Arthroscopy of the subtalar joint: An experimental approach. Arthroscopy 1985;1:53–7.
20. Lintz F, Guillard C, Colin F, et al. Safety and efficiency of a 2-portal lateral approach to arthroscopic subtalar arthrodesis: a cadaveric study. Arthroscopy 2013;29(7):1217–23.

21. Beimers L, Frey C, van Dijk CN. Arthroscopy of the posterior subtalar joint. Foot Ankle Clin N Am 2006;11:369–90.
22. William MM, Ferkel RD. Subtalar arthroscopy: indications, technique, and results. Arthroscopy 1998;14(4):373–81.
23. Cheng JC, Ferkel RD. The role of arthroscopy in ankle and subtalar degenerative joint disease. Clin Orthop Relat Res 1998;(349):65–72.
24. Lundeen RO. Arthroscopic fusion of the ankle and subtalar joint. Clin Podiatr Med Surg 1994;11:395–406.
25. Lee KB, Saltzman CL, Suh JS, et al. A posterior 3-portal arthroscopic approach for isolated subtalar arthrodesis. Arthroscopy 2008;24(11):1306–10.
26. Phisitkul P, Tochigi Y, Saltzman CL, et al. Arthroscopic visualization of the posterior subtalar joint in the prone position: a cadaver study. Arthroscopy 2006;22(5): 511–5.
27. Beals TC, Junko JT, Amendola A, et al. Minimally invasive distraction technique for prone posterior ankle and subtalar arthroscopy. Foot Ankle Int 2010;31:316–9.
28. Amendola A, Lee KB, Saltzman CL, et al. Technique and early experience with posterior arthroscopic subtalar arthrodesis. Foot Ankle Int 2007;28:298–302.
29. Mirmiran R, Wilde B, Nielson M. Retrospective analysis of the rate and interval to union for joint arthrodesis of the foot and ankle. J Foot Ankle Surg 2014;53:420–5.
30. Joveniaux P, Harisboure A, Ohl X, et al. Long-term results of in situ subtalar arthrodesis. Int Orthop 2010;34:1199–205.
31. Diezi C, Favre P, Vienne P. Primary isolated subtalar arthrodesis: outcome after 2 to 5 years followup. Foot Ankle Int 2008;29:1195–202.
32. Schepers T. The primary arthrodesis for severely comminuted intra-articular fractures of the calcaneus: a systematic review. J Foot Ankle Surg 2012;18:84–8.
33. Hungerer S, Trapp O, Augat P, et al. Posttraumatic arthrodesis of the subtalar joint—outcome in workers compensation and rates of non-union. J Foot Ankle Surg 2011;17:277–83.
34. Glanzmann MC, Sanhueza-Hernandez R. Arthroscopic subtalar arthrodesis for symptomatic osteoarthritis of the hindfoot: a prospective study of 41 cases. Foot Ankle Int 2007;28:2–7.
35. Scranton PE Jr. Comparison of open isolated subtalar arthrodesis with autogenous bone graft versus outpatient arthroscopic subtalar arthrodesis using injectable bone morphogenic protein-enhanced graft. Foot Ankle Int 1999;20:162–5.
36. Stegeman M, Louwerens JW, van der Woude JT, et al. Outcome after operative fusion of the tarsal joints: a systematic review. J Foot Ankle Surg 2014. [Epub ahead of print].
37. Nickisch F, Barg A, Saltzman CL, et al. Postoperative complications of posterior ankle and hindfoot arthroscopy. J Bone Joint Surg Am 2012;94:439–46.
38. Ebalard M, Le Henaff G, Sigonney G, et al. Risk of osteoarthritis secondary to partial or total arthrodesis of the subtalar and midtarsal joints after a minimum of 10 years. Orthop Traumatol Surg Res 2014;100:S231–7.

Distraction Subtalar Arthrodesis

J. Benjamin Jackson III, MD[a], Lance Jacobson, MD[b], Rahul Banerjee, MD[c],
Florian Nickisch, MD[b],*

KEYWORDS

- Arthritis • Arthrodesis • Calcaneus • Distraction • Fracture • Malunion • Osteotomy
- Subtalar

KEY POINTS

- Patients with calcaneal malunion can have significant functional limitations. They need a focused history, physical and radiographic examination.
- Selective injections can be useful in both locating the source of patient's pain and in preoperative discussions with the patient about expectations of pain relief after surgery.
- Adequate preparation of the subtalar joint and correction of the hindfoot deformity are important for a successful outcome.

INTRODUCTION

The calcaneus is the most commonly fractured tarsal bone. Calcaneal fractures account for approximately 60% to 70% of tarsal fractures and roughly 2% of all fractures.[1] The mechanism of injury is typically high-energy axial loading of the calcaneus, such as from a motor vehicle accident or a fall from height. These injuries have an important socioeconomic impact because 90% of patients sustaining calcaneal fractures are young and of working age.[2] Cotton and Henderson understood this in 1921 when they said, "The man who breaks his heel bone is done, so far as his industrial future is concerned."[3] For many patients, a calcaneal fracture is life altering and can be highly disabling. Displaced intra-articular calcaneal fractures frequently result in decreased hindfoot motion, persistent foot pain, and angular deformity.[4]

PATHOANATOMY OF CALCANEAL FRACTURE

Most calcaneal fractures are a result of axial loading. The lateral talar process wedges the calcaneus and forces the subtalar joint into eversion. As explained

Disclosures: The authors have nothing to disclose.
[a] Department of Orthopaedics, University of South Carolina, Columbia, SC, USA; [b] Department of Orthopaedics, University of Utah, Salt Lake City, UT, USA; [c] Department of Orthopaedics, Advent Orthopaedics, Plano, TX, USA
* Corresponding author. 590 Wakara Way, Salt Lake City, UT 84105.
E-mail address: florian.nickisch@hsc.utah.edu

by Böhler[5], this force causes a primary fracture line shearing the medial sustentaculum from the calcaneal tuberosity. It also leads to a secondary fracture line that occurs in the sagittal plane. These lines travel anteriorly and posteriorly, leading to posterior facet and anterior process comminution. The exit point of the secondary fracture lines varies and can exit the body of the calcaneus medially or laterally. Secondary fracture lines have been seen extending into the calcaneocuboid joint or splitting the anterior facet of the subtalar joint. Further impaction of the talus onto the calcaneus results in lateral displacement or blowout of the lateral calcaneal wall.[5]

The characteristic deformities seen in calcaneal fractures are a result of the primary and secondary fracture lines. Following fracture, the calcaneus is typically shortened and flattened as a result of the displacement through the primary fracture line. The sustentaculum tali usually remains with the talus, and the tuberosity displaces superolaterally. A recent study by Gitajn and colleagues[6] challenged the typical fracture pattern dogma because 44.3% of the calcaneus fractures they reviewed had sustentacular fractures. Only 11.7% were displaced but the investigators recommended evaluating the position of the sustentacular fragment to see whether this should be used as a landmark to anchor the fracture fixation. This short, flat appearance of the calcaneus is noted radiographically by a decrease in Böhler angle. It also causes the talus to rest in a more horizontal, dorsiflexed position that is seen radiographically as a decreased talar declination angle. The secondary fracture lines cause the additional deformities. The calcaneal tuberosity displaces into varus, leading to a varus heel position. In addition, the blowout of the lateral calcaneal wall results in a widened heel and subfibular impingement (**Fig. 1**). A recent study by Toussaint and colleagues[7] evaluated the rate of peroneal dislocation associated with 421 calcaneal fractures. A high rate (28.0%) of dislocated peroneals was noted and 89.8% of the dislocations were not noted on the radiology report. This study reaffirms the need for vigilance by surgeons treating these fractures to note the position of peroneal tendons on preoperative imaging.

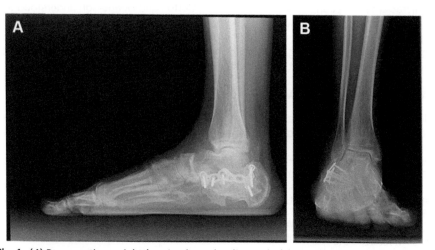

Fig. 1. (*A*) Preoperative weight-bearing lateral radiograph. (*B*) Preoperative weight-bearing mortise ankle radiograph. Note the overlap of the midfoot on the talus, indicating a flattened talus. This patient also has a widened heel and resultant subfibular impingement.

PATHOANATOMY OF CALCANEAL MALUNION

The resultant deformity dramatically alters the morphology of the calcaneus. If left untreated this change in morphology affects the function of the ankle and hindfoot, surrounding soft tissues, and joints. Sequelae include:

- Loss of height with anterior tibiotalar impingement
- Heel widening and subfibular impingement
- Calcaneocuboid joint arthrosis and impingement
- Varus heel
- Posttraumatic arthrosis of the subtalar joint
- Peroneal tendon disorder or dislocation
- Sural nerve disorder

LOSS OF HEIGHT AND ANTERIOR TIBIOTALAR IMPINGEMENT

A lateral radiograph of a healthy foot shows the Böhler angle.

An angle Böhler named the tuber-joint angle and described as an angle between the upper border of the calcaneal tuberosity and the line joining the highest point of the anterior process with the highest point of the posterior articular surface.[5] The normal angle varies from 25° to 40°. As a result of a calcaneal fracture, the calcaneus flattens, the Böhler angle decreases, and there is a loss of hindfoot height. These changes place the talus into a position that is more horizontal and dorsiflexed, which is seen radiographically as a change in the talar declination angle (**Fig. 2**).

This angle is again measured on the lateral radiograph of the foot. A line is drawn along the longitudinal axis of the talus, and a second line is drawn perpendicular to the first. A third line is drawn as a vertical line extending down from the intersection of the first two lines. The angle measured between the second and third lines is the talar declination. A decrease in this angle alters the mechanics of the tibiotalar joint. In the uninjured state the trapezoid shape of the talus allows normal ankle joint dorsiflexion and plantar flexion.[8] The more horizontal position of the talus may lead to wedging of the anterior aspect of the talar body into the ankle mortise, resulting in limited range of motion (ROM), anterior ankle impingement, and ankle arthrosis.[9]

In addition, a decrease in the height of the hindfoot shortens the lever arm for the gastrocnemius-soleus complex, which reduces the power that can be generated

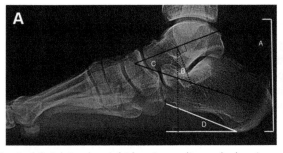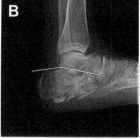

Fig. 2. (*A*) A lateral weight-bearing radiograph showing normal hindfoot measurements. Distance A represents calcaneal height. Angle B is talar declination angle; C, lateral talocalcaneal angle; D, calcaneal pitch. (*B*) Weight-bearing radiograph of a patient after a calcaneus fracture; note the common deformities that are present. They have a decreased Böhler angle (*white line*). They have a flattened talus and anterior impingement. The patient has also lost the calcaneal pitch and has a decreased calcaneal height, which decreases the lever arm of the triceps surae.

during the push-off phase of gait. Loss of height and heel widening can also lead to significant problems with shoe wear. With decreased hindfoot height, the malleoli are more likely to contact and rub on the shoe counter, which causes difficulty finding appropriate shoe wear and may lead to skin breakdown.

HEEL WIDENING AND SUBFIBULAR IMPINGEMENT

Lateral displacement of the lateral wall of the calcaneus results in heel widening. The displaced fragments may rest distal to the tip of the fibula. The resultant malunion can become a source of persistent pain. The pain can be a direct result of the bony abutment between the distal end of the fibula and the lateral blowout of the calcaneus. The pain may also represent entrapment and compression of the peroneal tendons between the bones, leading to tendinitis and tears.[10] In cases of more severe malunion there is residual lateral displacement of the calcaneus and this may cause the peroneal tendons may become sub- luxated or dislocated.[7,11]

VARUS HEEL

The tuberosity of the calcaneus typically displaces laterally and assumes a varus position; the result is overall varus hindfoot alignment. This condition has multiple implications for hindfoot function. Because the motion and function of the subtalar joint are coupled to the transverse tarsal joint, the new position of the hindfoot locks the transverse tarsal joint,[8] which may lead to a decrease in flexibility of the transverse tarsal joints during gait. The lack of flexibility decreases the natural shock-absorbing effect of the hindfoot. It can also lead to eccentric loading of the medial side of the ankle joint. In this way, varus hindfoot can accelerate wear and degeneration in multiple joints of the foot and ankle.

CALCANEOCUBOID JOINT IMPINGEMENT

As many as 48% of fractures involving the calcaneus also affect the calcaneocuboid joint.[12] Extension of the secondary fracture line into this joint may result in an anterolateral fragment. If this fragment is significantly displaced and remains malreduced, it may interfere with joint motion. This disruption of motion then results in calcaneocuboid joint impingement and less accommodation of the foot to the ground with normal gait.

POSTTRAUMATIC SUBTALAR ARTHROSIS

The injury and displacement of the subtalar joint as a result of the intra-articular calcaneal fracture may lead to posttraumatic arthrosis of the joint. In fractures of the talar neck, as little as 2 mm of displacement of the fracture was sufficient to significantly change the contact characteristics of the subtalar joint. These alterations in the contact of the joint lead to pain and degenerative arthritis.[13] It is presumed that displacement of a calcaneal fracture would have a similar effect on the subtalar joint. A relationship exists between displacement following calcaneal fracture and a poor clinical outcome. Outcomes are improved when there is anatomic reduction of the subtalar joint with anatomic restoration of the calcaneal width, height, length, and alignment.[14] Sanders and colleagues[15] also found that anatomic reduction improved joint function and diminished the likelihood of posttraumatic arthrosis. However, despite surgeons' best efforts, impaction of articular cartilage causes significant structural and metabolic changes that may predispose the involved cartilage to posttraumatic arthrosis.[16] This condition occurs regardless of anatomic reduction and thus may occur in calcaneal fractures that are nonsurgically managed, surgically treated with nonanatomic alignment, and even those that are anatomically reduced.

PREOPERATIVE EVALUATION
History and Physical Examination

Residual pain after fracture of the calcaneus can be present after surgical or nonsurgical management.[4,15,17–19]

Given the spectrum of residual disorders that can be present after a fracture of the calcaneus, the history and physical examination are key to determining the cause of pain or loss of function for each individual patient. Symptoms often correlate with the nature of the patient's original injury and a detailed history is important. The patients should be questioned about the:

- Original mechanism of injury
- Soft tissue injury (open vs closed)
- Initial treatment (surgical vs nonsurgical)
- If operatively treated, timing from injury to surgery

A detailed postoperative history should be obtained including:

- Any postoperative drainage/wound healing problems
- Use of antibiotics
- Additional procedures
- Resolution of initial postoperative pain
- Time from initial treatment to the onset of current symptoms

A social history of the patient should include occupation, lifestyle, functional demands, treatment expectations, and use of tobacco. Tobacco use has been shown to be a risk factor for nonunion with subtalar fusion.[20] Any medical comorbidities and current medication list should be reviewed and documented.

A detailed pain history should be taken including:

- Location
- Intensity
- Description
- Aggravating and alleviating factors

Identification of the correct source of symptoms is crucial for successful treatment. Physical examination of the foot and ankle should be comprehensive with careful attention paid to the patient's reported area of maximal pain.

The physical examination begins with a gait assessment noting any abnormalities by comparing the contralateral side, if uninjured. An antalgic gait, with a shortened stance phase, can be seen on the injured extremity and is common in patients with a symptomatic calcaneal malunion. The gross motion of the ankle and subtalar joint can also be observed during gait, particularly during the heel-strike and toe-off phases. Uneven weight distribution may even be noted during gait. If this is noted, the soles of the shoes can be examined for differences in wear pattern between the injured and uninjured limbs. Next, during the static standing examination, the physician can inspect the position of the ankle, hindfoot, and forefoot, in addition to observing for heel widening from both the front and back. If hindfoot abnormalities are noted, a Coleman block test can be performed to assess whether this deformity is forefoot or hindfoot driven.[21] Most often the hindfoot varus is an intrinsic deformity of the hindfoot caused by calcaneal varus malunion.

On seated examination the quality of the soft tissues can be noted, including the presence of any previous open wounds or surgical incisions. Next, passive and active ROM of the ankle, subtalar, and forefoot should be examined with attention paid to the patient's report of pain with motion. If the patient has limited ankle dorsiflexion, a Silfverskiöld test should be performed to determine whether the patient has an isolated gastrocnemius contracture versus a contracture of the triceps surae.[22] The average inversion of the hindfoot is 18° with 38° of eversion.[23] The ROM in each plane, any direction of limitation, and the percentage of motion should be compared with the contralateral side and recorded. We prefer to compare the subtalar motion as a percentage of the contralateral side, when uninjured, because measuring subtalar ROM can be unreliable, as noted by Buckley and Hunt.[24] In addition, the ROM of the toes should be evaluated along with any change in ROM with plantarflexion or dorsiflexion of the ankle. Changes in forefoot ROM could suggest neurologic injury, scarring from the sequelae of compartment syndrome, or tethering of the tendons that cross the hindfoot (flexor hallucis longus [FHL] or flexor digitorum longus). Palpation of the foot and ankle should try to illicit the patient's point of maximal tenderness.

A neurologic examination should include motor and strength testing of at least 1 muscle group for each of the 3 motor nerves in the foot. Sensation should be tested for each of the 5 sensory nerves of the foot and ankle with special attention paid to the sural nerve distribution on the lateral hindfoot. Any hyperesthesia, absence of perspiration, or lack of skin papillary lines should be noted because these can be sign of complex regional pain syndrome.

The history and physical examination can help to limit the differential diagnosis. The differential diagnosis based on the patient's report and examiner's observation of locations of maximal tenderness is discussed later.

Lateral Pain

The differential diagnosis for laterally based pain may be the result of:

- Subtalar arthrosis
- Peroneal tendon disorder
- Symptomatic hardware
- Calcaneofibular abutment
- Sural nerve disorder
- Calcaneocuboid arthrosis

The peroneal tendons can be initially assessed with direct palpation along their course to determine whether they are located in the retromalleolar grove and whether there is any tenderness to palpation. Then the examiner can ask the patient to actively evert the foot to assess strength, and subluxation or dislocation of the peroneal tendons. Depending on the severity of lateral calcaneal wall displacement or calcaneofibular abutment, a patient can have peroneal disorder ranging from peroneal tenosynovitis to scarring to incomplete or complete tears of the peroneal tendons.[10,11] Subluxation or dislocation of the tendons can occur because of the reduction of size in the subfibular space that the tendons occupy or because of the attenuation of the superior peroneal retinaculum.[11]

Tenderness of the sinus tarsi can help distinguish subtalar arthrosis from calcaneocuboid arthrosis, which has an area of tenderness that is more inferior and slightly more distal. Calcaneocuboid arthrosis can occur as frequently as subtalar arthrosis, but is less commonly symptomatic.[25]

If the patient was treated operatively with a lateral approach and hardware placement the retained hardware can be a source of pain. The fullness from any residual edema combined with retained hardware can cause difficultly with shoe wear. Any prominent hardware that has failed and/or backed out can cause pain. Palpation along the hardware may help distinguish the portion that is most symptomatic.

Both surgically and conservatively managed patients can have sural nerve disorder. Patients with sural nerve disorder may describe symptoms of pain at rest, paresthesia, anesthesia, or hyperesthesia along the lateral border of the heel that may extend into the foot. Patients with hyperesthesia may describe intolerance to any material touching the foot, or difficultly with sock or shoe wear. These patients should be evaluated for complex regional pain syndrome. A Tinel test may be performed by tapping along the course of the sural nerve to examine for reproduction of pain. The location and density of any paresthesia or anesthesia should be documented. The presence of abnormal sensation can be determined with use of a 5.07 Semmes-Weinstein monofilament compared with published controls.[26]

Anterior Pain

Dorsal foot or anterior ankle pain is common after calcaneal fracture malunion. Lindsay and Dewar found that 22% to 35% of their patients with pain after calcaneal fracture had pain in the ankle.[19] This pain is most often caused by anterior ankle impingement from loss of calcaneal height that then leads to flattening of the talus and loss of talar declination. The altered biomechanics can lead to anterior ankle impingement and decreased ankle dorsiflexion.[27] Patients with complaints of anterior pain should be examined for active and passive ROM of the ankle. Dorsiflexion is usually limited in these patients, which can be caused by bony impingement, as described earlier, or by soft tissue contracture. The examiner should measure dorsiflexion with the knee flexed and extended to detect the effect of gastrocnemius or triceps surae on any restriction to dorsiflexion.[22]

Plantar Pain

Plantar or heel pain is common after a severe calcaneus fracture, being present in 26% to 38% of patients.[19] Plantar pain can have a large differential, with some causes related to the initial injury and others related to the residual deformity. The initial injury can damage the soft tissues around the calcaneus or direct injury can damage the heel pad. The damage to the soft tissues or heel pad can cause chronic and, at times, debilitating plantar pain. Clinicians can examine for atrophy of the heel pad and focal areas of tenderness to palpation versus generalized heel pain. Focal areas of tenderness to palpation can be from residual deformity or malunion of the calcaneus. The palpated prominences can be correlated with those seen on radiographs.

Medial Pain

The close relationship of the FHL tendon and the medial wall of the calcaneus make even small residual deformities of this side of the calcaneus potentially pathologic. Medial wall deformity can cause scarring and tethering of the FHL, which can lead to a progression of symptoms from pain with passive ROM of the great toe to loss of ROM to a flexible or fixed contracture of the first metatarsophalangeal or interphalangeal joint. The contracture, or cock-up deformity, may become more flexible with ankle plantar flexion if it is caused by FHL tethering.

More severe medial wall deformities or valgus malunion of the calcaneal tuberosity may cause tarsal tunnel syndrome. The patient may describe vague medial-sided foot pain. A Tinel test along the tibial nerve can help distinguish tarsal tunnel syndrome from plantar fasciitis. The patient's foot can be passively dorsiflexed and everted to see whether this exacerbates the patient's symptoms.

IMAGING STUDIES

To evaluate patients with calcaneal malunion we obtain weight-bearing anteroposte-rior (AP), lateral, and lateral column oblique views of the foot along with axial (Harris view)[28] and hindfoot alignment roentograms.[29] Contralateral views can be obtained as indicated to determine the patient's normal alignment. Radiographs should be examined for arthrosis of the subtalar, ankle, and calcaneocuboid joints. Subfibular impingement can be seen on the weight-bearing mortise view. Anterior ankle impinge-ment is best seen on the lateral film. The measurement of certain established angles and distances can be helpful in preoperative planning.

The Böhler angle is measured on lateral radiographs and has been shown to be an important predictor of patient outcome after calcaneus fracture (see **Fig. 2**).[30] Resto-ration of the calcaneal height is important in surgical reconstruction of the malunited calcaneus.

The heel width can be assessed on the axial or Harris heel views (**Fig. 3**).[28] The lateral wall blowout with severe fracture often leads to increased heel width, which can lead to pain and difficultly with shoe wear. From this radiograph clinicians can evaluate for varus of valgus malalignment; however, the hindfoot alignment view allows a more accurate assessment of alignment.[31]

The hindfoot alignment view can be used to determine any residual varus or valgus of the hindfoot by measuring the tibiocalcaneal displacement (**Fig. 4**).[29]

Restoration of the normal alignment of the tibiotalar-calcaneal axis can help restore more normal biomechanics of the hindfoot for the patient.

Myerson and Quill[32] measured the loss of height of the calcaneus and loss of talar declination angles. They found that loss of more than 8 mm of calcaneal height, compared with the uninjured side, and a talar declination angle of less than 20° was an indication for bone-block arthrodesis.[32] Other studies have examined the

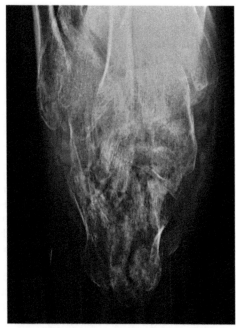

Fig. 3. The Harris, or axial, view is used to assess both heel width and varus malalignment.

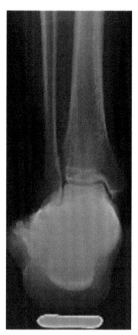

Fig. 4. A hindfoot alignment view can also be helpful for assessing the hindfoot's relationship to the tibia and ankle.

correlation of these measurements and patient outcomes, as measured by American Orthopaedic Foot and Ankle Society (AOFAS) score.[33,34]

Advanced imaging can be extremely helpful in the assessment of patients with severe or complex deformities. Easley and colleagues[35] suggested that computer-assisted three-dimensional preoperative planning may help facilitate surgery. We obtain a computed tomography (CT) scan on every patient that is being considered for distraction arthrodesis.

CT scans are useful for:

- Assessing the three-dimensional deformity
- Evaluating for fracture healing
- Assessing for subtalar, calcaneocuboid arthrosis
- Evaluating peroneal tendon position
- Measuring the shortening of the hindfoot

DIAGNOSTIC INJECTIONS

As discussed earlier, the differential can be extensive and it can be difficult to elucidate the specific cause of the pain. When the exact source of pain is unclear, selective diagnostic injections can be particularly helpful. Myerson and Quill[32] found that selective injection of patients with pain after calcaneus fracture was a helpful diagnostic tool. Injection of 1% Xylocaine or 0.5% bupivacaine was helpful in diagnosing the correct cause of the pain in 21 of 24 patients who were injected.[32] Some clinicians use a combination of local anesthetic (eg, 0.5% bupivacaine) and a corticosteroid for both diagnostic and therapeutic benefit in these patients. Chu and colleagues[36] studied the use of a single injection of 0.5% bupivacaine on articular cartilage in a rat knee model and found that it did not reduce the cartilage tissue viability at 6 months.

It has been recommended that diagnostic selective injections be performed with the assistance of fluoroscopic guidance and contrast material.[37] Kirk and colleagues[37] found that foot and ankle–trained surgeons were able to place an injection in the posterior subtalar joint in 96.6% of cadaveric specimens. However, because these injections can be a critical step in the diagnostic algorithm and they had injections with both extra-articular and peroneal sheath extravasation, they recommended that these injections be performed under fluoroscopic guidance.

We use radiologists with musculoskeletal training for injections. They perform injections of the peroneal tendon sheath, sural nerve, tibial nerve, subtalar, ankle, or calcaneocuboid joints with fluoroscopic guidance and contrast to enhance their accuracy.

MANAGEMENT

Conservative management, including activity modification, shoe wear modification, rocker-bottom shoes, orthoses, injections, functional rehabilitation, bracing, and pain medications are the mainstays of initial treatment. If these modalities are unsuccessful, custom orthoses with additional heel cushioning and specific wedges that address hindfoot malalignment or deformity can be helpful. The final step in conservative management, because of its cumbersome nature, is typically a double-upright or Arizona brace (Arizona Inc, Mesa, AZ). This brace reduces the motion of the ankle and subtalar joints and can provide some pain relief and patient satisfaction.

Patients who fail these conservative measures and are medically fit are candidates for surgical intervention. The surgical options include lateral wall decompression, in situ subtalar arthrodesis, subtalar distraction arthrodesis, corrective calcaneal osteotomy with arthrodesis, and triple arthrodesis. This article only discusses in detail our preferred technique for subtalar distraction arthrodesis.

AUTHORS' PREFERRED TECHNIQUE

Patients who are considered for this reconstructive technique have a calcaneal malunion with symptomatic subtalar arthritis and anterior ankle impingement caused by a loss of calcaneal height and a horizontal talus. Radiographically these patients have a decreased talar declination angle, loss of Böhler angle, subtalar joint arthrosis, and anterior ankle joint impingement with the corresponding osteophytes on the talus or tibia.[38] We use criteria similar to those proposed by Myerson and Quill.[32] They found that loss of more than 8 mm of calcaneal height, compared with the uninjured side, and a talar declination angle of less than 20° was an indication for bone-block arthrodesis.[32] Other studies have found that using these criteria can lead to improve patient outcomes as measured by the AOFAS score.[33,34]

The importance of preoperative determination, as described in detail earlier, of the exact cause of a patient's pain or functional limitation is critical in determining the correct operation for a patient. Preoperative weight-bearing radiographs and a CT scan help assess the deformity and the amount of correction that is needed. Lateral wall widening, adjacent joint arthrosis, and the peroneal tendons, in the soft tissue windows, can be assessed with CT imaging. However, the imaging findings must be correlated with the patient's physical examination findings to determine whether distraction or in situ arthrodesis is indicated.[33]

Patients are counseled preoperatively about the importance of tobacco cessation and its impact on subtalar arthrodesis.[20,39] They are also counseled on the postoperative recovery and prolonged period of non–weight bearing. Personal and family history risk factors for deep venous thrombosis and pulmonary embolism are assessed.

The operative approach is influenced by any previous incisions. Some investigators have recommended the extensile lateral approach, particularly if the patient has retained hardware.[9,40] Some have reported increased wound complications, particularly in the horizontal limb, and this was hypothesized to be caused by increased wound tension after the distraction arthrodesis.[41] The wound infections in this series were superficial and resolved with oral antibiotics alone.[41] Amendola and Lammens[42] recommended the modified Kocher approach, whereas others use the approach described by Gallie.[43] We routinely use the Gallie[43] longitudinal posterolateral approach.

- We use regional anesthesia with a popliteal block along with general anesthesia. A popliteal catheter can be placed for approximately 36 hours of postoperative pain relief.
- The patient is placed in either the lateral decubitus position with a beanbag or prone.
- A thigh tourniquet is placed.
- The ipsilateral anterior or posterior iliac crest and the operative leg from the knee down are prepped and draped.
- Blunt dissection is taken down to the deep crural fascia with care taken to avoid the sural nerve.
- After the deep crural fascia is incised, the interval between the FHL and peroneus longus tendons is developed.
- If retained hardware is present we remove it at this stage of the operation. Any hardware that is not directly visualized from the approach is removed percutaneously with the assistance of fluoroscopy.
- Occasionally, a separate sinus tarsi incision is needed to assist in hardware removal.
- A full-thickness lateral soft tissue flap can be developed, elevating the soft tissues from the lateral wall of the calcaneus (or the plate and screws) with a Cobb or other periosteal elevator.
- After hardware removal we then inspect the heel width and, if needed, perform a lateral wall decompression from posterior to anterior with a 12-mm or 19-mm (0.5-inch or 0.75-inch) osteotome. The excised bone is saved for later use as bone graft.
- With the subtalar joints exposed, the common deformity of the talar body depressed into the calcaneus can be noted.
- Next, a Hintermann retractor or femoral distractor is placed percutaneously from the tibia to the calcaneus on the medial side of the leg in order to prevent varus malalignment.
- If distraction of the subtalar joint is difficult, then the surgeon should assess for gastrocnemius or Achilles tendon contracture.
- If the contracture is isolated to the gastrocnemius we perform a recession through a separate posteromedial incision on the calf, as described by Baumann and Koch.[44]
- If we find a combined contracture of the triceps surae we perform a Hoke percutaneous lengthening.[45]
- After the joint is adequately distracted, the joint surfaces are cleaned of any residual cartilage and prepared for arthrodesis.
- In cases of severe or long-standing deformity, medial-sided contracture may prevent complete correction. This deformity can be released with an angled curette or periosteal elevator from the lateral side.

- Care must be taken to avoid injury to the structures on the posteromedial side of the hindfoot, including the neurovascular bundle. Lateral fluoroscopy is necessary to determine the amount of distraction that is needed for complete correction of the deformity. We use the lateral technique to ensure restoration of talar declination angle. Normal talar declination can be seen in **Fig. 2**A.
- After the deformity is fully corrected, the size of the graft that is needed can be assessed.
- We use anterior or posterior iliac crest autograft, depending on the size needed. A tricortical graft is harvested with the technique described by Hansen.[46]
- When a single large bone block is used we place it slightly medially in order to prevent varus.[46]
- If there is significant sagittal plane deformity we use 2 separate grafts placed side by side in order to correct varus/valgus malalignment.[47]
- After the graft is selected it is shaped into a trapezoid with the lateral aspect of the wedge being slightly shorter than the medial side to avoid varus malalignment.
- Distraction is released and the varus/valgus correction is assessed clinically and fluoroscopically.
- In some cases the tuber is displaced so far laterally that a medializing osteotomy is also needed. The need for this additional osteotomy is best evaluated on the axial heel view.
- If the correction is acceptable then any residual voids are filled with cancellous autograft, or excised lateral wall autograft.
- Fixation of the subtalar joint is done using 6.5-mm or 7.3-mm cannulated screws. Multiple different configurations have been described for screw placement.[20,48,49]
- We usually place 2 screws percutaneously from the posterior to inferior calcaneal tuber, 1 into the talar body and 1 into the talar neck.
- The first screw is a partially threaded preferably a 7.3-mm screw placed into the neck of the talus (pulling the neck plantarly). The second screw is preferably a fully threaded 7.3-mm screw placed into the talar body. The fully threaded screw is used to prevent collapse of the graft and subtalar joint.
- Adequate correction is confirmed again with AP and mortise fluoroscopic images of the ankle along with lateral and AP images of the foot and axial view of the heel.
- The wounds are closed in layers and a plaster splint is applied with the patient in a plantigrade position with neutral sagittal alignment (**Fig. 5**).

POSTOPERATIVE CARE

The patient is made non–weight bearing and is in a cast or splint for 6 to 8 weeks. If radiographs at that time are acceptable, then the patient is placed into a walking boot and begins a progressive weight-bearing regimen that is supervised by physical therapy. Our regimen is an initial 11 kg (25 lb) of weight on the operative extremity and progression by 11 kg every 3 to 4 days until full weight bearing. Once the patient can fully weight bear in the walking boot without pain and there are adequate radiographic signs of healing on the 12-week postoperative radiographs, the patient is then allowed to transition, as swelling allows, into a regular shoe.

PUBLISHED RESULTS

Several studies have evaluated patient outcomes following subtalar distraction bone-block arthrodesis for nonunion. Gallie[43] was the first to describe a posterior approach

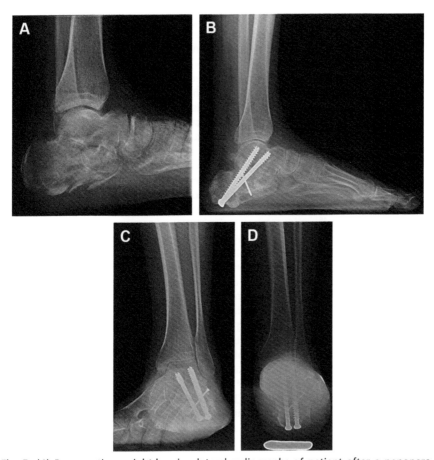

Fig. 5. (A) Preoperative weight-bearing lateral radiographs of patient after a nonopera-tively managed calcaneus fracture. The typical findings of a flattened talus and loss of calca-neal height can been seen. Postoperative lateral (B), ankle mortise (C), and hindfoot (D) alignment views after subtalar distraction bone-block arthrodesis. Note the improve-ment in calcaneal height and the improved talar declination angle.

to subtalar joint arthrodesis with insertion of bone-block allograft from the tibia. He did this without fixation in 1943. He performed this method on 50 patients over 6 years and reported successful results. Note was made of only 1 failed fusion during this time.[43] Carr and colleagues[41] modified the procedure and published their outcomes. This report on 16 feet was done at a mean follow-up period of 19 months. These patients all had subtalar fusion with distraction and insertion of a bone block. Results were re-ported to be satisfactory in 13 of the 16 feet. Radiographic analysis for tibiotalar impingement and lateral talocalcaneal and talonavicular subluxation postoperatively showed improvement to a normal range. Their reported complications included nonunion, sural nerve neuroma, infection, and painful retained hardware.

A larger series from Bednarz and colleagues[39] retrospectively reviewed 29 feet in 28 patients who underwent subtalar distraction bone arthrodesis found a significant improvement in AOFAS scores (P<.0001). They also found a significant improvement in measured radiographic parameters including hindfoot height, lateral talocalcaneal angle, and lateral talar declination angle. They also noted a significant risk of smoking on nonunion. Ninety percent of their patients reported satisfaction with surgery. They reported 4 nonunions, all in smokers, and 2 varus malunions. They also had 1 metatarsal stress fracture and 1 medial plantar nerve anesthesia that were attributed to the procedure.

Trnka and colleagues[49] performed a retrospective analysis of the results of subtalar bone-block distraction arthrodesis. A total of 35 patients (37 feet) were examined at a mean follow-up period of 70 months. Union rate following arthrodesis was 86.5% (32 of 37) and 29 of the 31 (93.5%) patients who achieved arthrodesis were satisfied with the outcome. AOFAS ankle hindfoot scores significantly improved from 22.1 before the operation to 68.9 at follow-up. Complications included nonunion, avascular necrosis of the talus or calcaneus, sural neuralgia, infection, and prominent hardware. Comparable results were seen in several other studies. Amendola and Lammens[42] showed that, according to a visual analogue scale, 11 of 15 patients were satisfied with their outcomes following subtalar arthrodesis using interposition iliac crest bone graft. Chan and Alexander[48] also reported a significant improvement in AOFAS hindfoot scores from less than 50 preoperatively to a mean of 75 following surgery.

Similar results were seen by Rammelt and colleagues[9] who studied a total of 31 patients (26 men and 5 women) who underwent unilateral subtalar distraction bone-block arthrodesis for posttraumatic subtalar arthritis secondary to calcaneal malunion. The patients were examined at 6 and 12 weeks postoperatively. Patients were then contacted after a minimum of 2 years postoperatively. Patients were evaluated prospectively with regard to functional scoring (using the AOFAS Ankle Hindfoot Scale) and clinical and radiological findings. Postoperative complications were seen in 12.9% of patients and included dislocation of the bone block, soft tissue infection, painful plantar exostosis, and allergic local skin reaction. All patients had a subjectively and clinically stable hindfoot and all went on to solid union of the arthrodesis. In all, 93.6% were satisfied with the result. The mean AOFAS hindfoot score significantly improved from 23.5 to 73.2. Radiographic evaluation showed that after arthrodesis there was significant improvement in alignment despite correction not reaching the measurements found on the unaffected side.

A more recent retrospective study analyzed 22 consecutive patients who underwent posterior bone-block subtalar joint arthrodesis with a minimum follow-up period of 12 months. Of these 22 patients, 21 (95.5%) went on to radiographic and clinical fusion. Radiographic data found a statistically significant improvement in heel height postoperatively compared with preoperative radiographs. Complications included nonunion, wound dehiscence, varus malunion, and painful retained hardware.[50]

SUMMARY

Patients with calcaneal malunion can have significant functional limitations. These patients need a focused history and physical examination along with a radiographic evaluation. It is important to locate the patient's point of maximal tenderness. Selective injections can be useful in locating the cause of the patient's pain and in preoperative discussions with the patient about expectations of pain relief after surgery. Adequate preparation of the subtalar joint and correction of the hindfoot deformity are important for a successful outcome. Studies of this procedure indicate that most patients have significant preoperative limitations but have a reasonable improvement after surgery.

REFERENCES

1. O'Connell F, Mital MA, Rowe CR. Evaluation of modern management of fractures of the os calcis. Clin Orthop Relat Res 1972;83:214–23.

2. Tanke GM. Fractures of the calcaneus. A review of the literature together with some observations on methods of treatment. Acta Chir Scand Suppl 1982;505: 1–103.
3. Cotton FJ. Old os calcis fractures. Ann Surg 1921;74:294–303.
4. Radnay CS, Clare MP, Sanders RW. Subtalar fusion after displaced intra-articular calcaneal fractures: does initial operative treatment matter? J Bone Joint Surg Am 2009;91:541–6.
5. Lorenz B. Diagnosis, pathology, and treatment of fractures of the os calcis. J Bone Joint Surg Am 1931;13(1):75–89.
6. Gitajn IL, Abousayed M, Toussaint RJ, et al. Anatomic alignment and integrity of the sustentaculum tali in intra-articular calcaneal fractures: is the sustentaculum tali truly constant? J Bone Joint Surg Am 2014;96:1000–5.
7. Toussaint RJ, Lin D, Ehrlichman LK, et al. Peroneal tendon displacement accompanying intra-articular calcaneal fractures. J Bone Joint Surg Am 2014; 96:310–5.
8. Sarrafian SK. Sarrafian's anatomy of the foot and ankle: descriptive, topographical, functional. In: Kelikian AS, Sarrafian SK, editors. Philadelphia: Wolters Kluwer Health/Lippincott Williams & Wilkins; 2011. p. 62–9.
9. Rammelt S, Grass R, Zawadski T, et al. Foot function after subtalar distraction bone-block arthrodesis. A prospective study. J Bone Joint Surg Br 2004;86: 659–68.
10. Isbister JF. Calcaneo-fibular abutment following crush fracture of the calcaneus. J Bone Joint Surg Br 1974;56:274–8.
11. Rosenberg ZS, Feldman F, Singson RD, et al. Peroneal tendon injury associated with calcaneal fractures: CT findings. AJR Am J Roentgenol 1987;149:125–9.
12. Silhanek AD, Ramdass R, Lombardi CM. The effect of primary fracture line location on the pattern and severity of intraarticular calcaneal fractures: a retrospective radiographic study. J Foot Ankle Surg 2006;45:211–9.
13. Sangeorzan BJ, Wagner UA, Harrington RM, et al. Contact characteristics of the subtalar joint: the effect of talar neck misalignment. J Orthop Res 1992;10:544–51.
14. Paley D, Hall H. Intra-articular fractures of the calcaneus. A critical analysis of results and prognostic factors. J Bone Joint Surg Am 1993;75:342–54.
15. Sanders R, Fortin P, DiPasquale T, et al. Operative treatment in 120 displaced intraarticular calcaneal fractures. Results using a prognostic computed tomography scan classification. Clin Orthop Relat Res 1993;(290):87–95.
16. Catalano LW, Cole RJ, Gelberman RH, et al. Displaced intra-articular fractures of the distal aspect of the radius. Long-term results in young adults after open reduction and internal fixation. J Bone Joint Surg Am 1997;79:1290–302.
17. Crosby LA, Fitzgibbons T. Intraarticular calcaneal fractures. Results of closed treatment. Clin Orthop Relat Res 1993;(290):47–54.
18. Stephens HM, Sanders R. Calcaneal malunions: results of a prognostic computed tomography classification system. Foot Ankle Int 1996;17:395–401.
19. Lindsay WR, Dewar FP. Fractures of the os calcis. Am J Surg 1958;95:555–76.
20. Easley ME, Trnka HJ, Schon LC, et al. Isolated subtalar arthrodesis. J Bone Joint Surg Am 2000;82:613–24.
21. Coleman SS, Chesnut WJ. A simple test for hindfoot flexibility in the cavovarus foot. Clin Orthop Relat Res 1977;(123):60–2.
22. Silfverskiöld N. Reduction of the uncrossed two-joints muscles of the leg to one-joint muscles in spastic conditions. Acta Chir Scand 1924;56:1923–4.
23. Roaas A, Andersson GB. Normal range of motion of the hip, knee and ankle joints in male subjects, 30-40 years of age. Acta Orthop Scand 1982;53:205–8.

24. Buckley RE, Hunt DV. Reliability of clinical measurement of subtalar joint movement. Foot Ankle Int 1997;18:229–32.

25. Banerjee R, Saltzman C, Anderson RB, et al. Management of calcaneal malunion. J Am Acad Orthop Surg 2011;19:27–36.

26. Jeng C, Michelson J, Mizel M. Sensory thresholds of normal human feet. Foot Ankle Int 2000;21:501–4.

27. Kitaoka HB, Schaap EJ, Chao EY, et al. Displaced intra-articular fractures of the calcaneus treated non-operatively. Clinical results and analysis of motion and ground-reaction and temporal forces. J Bone Joint Surg Am 1994;76:1531–40.

28. Harris RI, Beath T. Etiology of peroneal spastic flat foot. J Bone Joint Surg Br 1948;30B:624–34.

29. Saltzman CL, el-Khoury GY. The hindfoot alignment view. Foot Ankle Int 1995;16: 572–6.

30. Csizy M, Buckley R, Tough S, et al. Displaced intra-articular calcaneal fractures: variables predicting late subtalar fusion. J Orthop Trauma 2003;17:106–12.

31. Barg A, Harris MD, Henninger HB, et al. Medial distal tibial angle: comparison between weightbearing mortise view and hindfoot alignment view. Foot Ankle Int 2012;33:655–61.

32. Myerson M, Quill GE. Late complications of fractures of the calcaneus. J Bone Joint Surg Am 1993;75:331–41.

33. Chandler JT, Bonar SK, Anderson RB, et al. Results of in situ subtalar arthrodesis for late sequelae of calcaneus fractures. Foot Ankle Int 1999;20:18–24.

34. Flemister AS, Infante AF, Sanders RW, et al. Subtalar arthrodesis for complications of intra-articular calcaneal fractures. Foot Ankle Int 2000;21:392–9.

35. Easley M, Chuckpaiwong B, Cooperman N, et al. Computer-assisted surgery for subtalar arthrodesis. A study in cadavers. J Bone Joint Surg Am 2008;90: 1628–36.

36. Chu CR, Coyle CH, Chu CT, et al. In vivo effects of single intra-articular injection of 0.5% bupivacaine on articular cartilage. J Bone Joint Surg Am 2010;92:599–608.

37. Kirk KL, Campbell JT, Guyton GP, et al. Accuracy of posterior subtalar joint injection without fluoroscopy. Clin Orthop Relat Res 2008;466:2856–60.

38. Romash MM. Reconstructive osteotomy of the calcaneus with subtalar arthrodesis for malunited calcaneal fractures. Clin Orthop Relat Res 1993;(290):157–67.

39. Bednarz PA, Beals TC, Manoli A. Subtalar distraction bone block fusion: an assessment of outcome. Foot Ankle Int 1997;18:785–91.

40. Clare MP, Lee WE, Sanders RW. Intermediate to long-term results of a treatment protocol for calcaneal fracture malunions. J Bone Joint Surg Am 2005;87:963–73.

41. Carr JB, Hansen ST, Benirschke SK. Subtalar distraction bone block fusion for late complications of os calcis fractures. Foot Ankle 1988;9:81–6.

42. Amendola A, Lammens P. Subtalar arthrodesis using interposition iliac crest bone graft after calcaneal fracture. Foot Ankle Int 1996;17:608–14.

43. Gallie WE. Subastragalar arthrodesis in fractures of the os calcis. J Bone Joint Surg Am 1943;25:731–6.

44. Baumann JU, Koch HG. Ventrale aponeurotische Verlängerung des Musculus gastrocnemius. Oper Orthop Traumatol 1989;1:254–8.

45. Hatt RN, Lamphier TA. Triple hemisection: a simplified procedure for lengthening the Achilles tendon. N Engl J Med 1947;236:166–9.

46. Hansen ST. Functional reconstruction of the foot and ankle. Lippincott Williams & Wilkins; 2000.

47. Zwipp H, Rammelt S. Posttraumatic deformity correction at the foot. Zentralbl Chir 2003;128:218–26 [in German].

48. Chan SC, Alexander IJ. Subtalar arthrodesis with interposition tricortical iliac crest graft for late pain and deformity after calcaneus fracture. Foot Ankle Int 1997;18:613–5.
49. Trnka HJ, Easley ME, Lam PW, et al. Subtalar distraction bone block arthrodesis. J Bone Joint Surg Br 2001;83:849–54.
50. Pollard JD, Schuberth JM. Posterior bone block distraction arthrodesis of the subtalar joint: a review of 22 cases. J Foot Ankle Surg 2008;47:191–8.

Index

Note: Page numbers of article titles are in **boldface** type.

Foot Ankle Clin N Am 20 (2015) 353–380
http://dx.doi.org/10.1016/S1083-7515(15)00044-3
1083-7515/15/$ – see front matter © 2015 Elsevier Inc. All rights reserved.

Moving?

Make sure your subscription moves with you!

To notify us of your new address, find your **Clinics Account Number** (located on your mailing label above your name), and contact customer service at:

Email: journalscustomerservice-usa@elsevier.com

800-654-2452 (subscribers in the U.S. & Canada)
314-447-8871 (subscribers outside of the U.S. & Canada)

Fax number: 314-447-8029

Elsevier Health Sciences Division
Subscription Customer Service
3251 Riverport Lane
Maryland Heights, MO 63043

*To ensure uninterrupted delivery of your subscription, please notify us at least 4 weeks in advance of move.